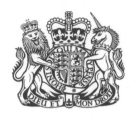

Valuing People

A New Strategy for Learning Disability for the 21st Century

A White Paper

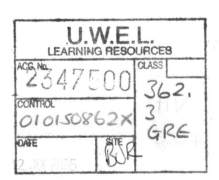
Presented to Parliament by the
Secretary of State for Health by
Command of Her Majesty
March 2001

Cm 5086   £15.90

CONTENTS

FOREWORD BY THE
PRIME MINISTER

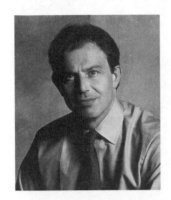

People with learning disabilities can lead full and rewarding lives as many already do. But others find themselves pushed to the margins of our society. And almost all encounter prejudice, bullying, insensitive treatment and discrimination at some time in their lives.

Such prejudice and discrimination – no less hurtful for often being unintentional – has a very damaging impact. It leads to your world becoming smaller, opportunities more limited, a withdrawal from wider society so time is spent only with family, carers or other people with learning disabilities.

What's also a real cause for concern and anxiety is that many parents of learning disabled children face difficulties in finding the right care, health services, education and leisure opportunities for their sons and daughters. At best, they can feel obstacles are constantly put in their way by society. At worst, they feel abandoned by the rest of us.

We have to change this situation if we are to achieve our goal of a modern society in which everyone is valued and has the chance to play their full part. There has been progress – often through the efforts of families, voluntary organisations and people with learning disabilities themselves. But a great deal more needs to be done.

This White Paper sets out this Government's commitment to improving the life chances of people with learning disabilities. It shows how we will meet this commitment by working closely with local councils, the health service, voluntary organisations and most importantly with people with learning disabilities and their families to provide new opportunities for those with learning disabilities to lead full and active lives.

I know the publication of a White Paper, however good its proposals, does not itself solve problems. The challenge for us all is to deliver the vision set out in this document so the lives of many thousands of people with learning disabilities will be brighter and more fulfilling. It is a challenge I am determined this Government will meet.

Tony Blair

EXECUTIVE SUMMARY

People with learning disabilities are amongst the most vulnerable and socially excluded in our society. Very few have jobs, live in their own homes or have choice over who cares for them. This needs to change: people with learning disabilities must no longer be marginalised or excluded. *Valuing People* sets out how the Government will provide new opportunities for children and adults with learning disabilities and their families to live full and independent lives as part of their local communities.

Where we are today

Problems and Challenges

There are about 210,000 people with severe learning disabilities in England, and about 1.2 million with a mild or moderate disability. Health and social services expenditure on services for adults with learning disabilities stands at around £3 billion. In the 30 years since the last White Paper *Better Services for the Mentally Handicapped*, progress has been made in closing large institutions and developing services in the community, but more needs to be done. There are major problems, including:

- Poorly co-ordinated services for **families with disabled children especially for those with severely disabled children;**

- Poor planning for **young disabled people at the point of transition into adulthood;**

- Insufficient support for **carers, particularly for those caring for people with complex needs;**

- People with learning disabilities often have little **choice or control** over many aspects of their lives;

- Substantial **health care** needs of people with learning disabilities are often unmet;

- **Housing choice** is limited;

- **Day services** are often not tailored to the needs and abilities of the individual;

- Limited opportunities for **employment;**

- The needs of **people from minority ethnic communities** are often overlooked;

- **Inconsistency in expenditure and service delivery**; and

- Few examples of real **partnership** between health and social care or involving people with learning disabilities and carers.

The New Vision

- Four key principles of **Rights, Independence, Choice, Inclusion** lie at the heart of the Government's proposals. Legislation which confers rights on all citizens, including the Human Rights Act 1998 and the Disability Discrimination Act 1995, applies equally to all people with learning disabilities, and the Disability Rights Commission will work for people with learning disabilities.

- New national objectives for services for people with learning disabilities, supported by new targets and performance indicators, to provide clear direction for local agencies

- A new **Learning Disability Development Fund of up to £50 million per annum from April 2002**: £20 million capital and up to £30 million revenue. The revenue element of the Development Fund will be created from within old long-stay health funding as it is released over time. The Development Fund will be targeted on the key priorities of the White Paper, including modernising day centres, enabling people to move from long-stay hospitals to more appropriate accommodation in the community, developing supported living approaches for people living with older carers, developing specialist local services for people with severe challenging behaviour and developing integrated facilities for children with severe disabilities and complex needs. The Development Fund will be made available subject to the condition that resources may only be used where they are deployed as pooled funds under the Health Act flexibilities.

- A new central **Implementation Support Fund of £2.3 million a year for the next 3 years** that will be used to fund a range of developments including advocacy and a new national information centre and help line.

Better life chances for people with learning disabilities

Disabled Children and Young People

- Learning disabled children and their families face many barriers to full participation in society. The Government's objective is to ensure that disabled children gain maximum life chance benefits from educational opportunities, health and social care while living with their families or in other appropriate settings.

- To achieve this we will ensure that learning disabled children and their families are an integral part of the Quality Protects programme, the Department for Education and Employment's Special Educational Needs Programme of Action and the Connexions Service. Disabled children will be a priority group under the Quality Protects programme with £60 million over the next three years earmarked to provide better support. The Schools Access Initiative will provide funds to improve accessibility of mainstream schools and the Standards Fund will be used to improve provision for children with special educational needs.

- Transition from childhood to adulthood can be a particularly difficult process for both disabled children and their parents/carers. Our objective is to ensure continuity of care and support and equality of opportunity for young people and their families so that as many learning disabled young people as possible take part in education, training, or employment. The Connexions Service will provide new help and advice to disabled young people as they move into adult life.

More Choice and Control for People with Learning Disabilities

- People with learning disabilities have little control over their lives, few receive direct payments, advocacy services are underdeveloped and people with learning disabilities are often not central to the planning process. The Government's objective is to enable people with learning disabilities to have as much choice and control as possible over their lives and the services and support they receive.

- To achieve this, we are investing at least **£1.3 million a year for the next 3 years to develop advocacy services** for people with learning disabilities in partnership with the voluntary sector. We are extending eligibility for direct payments through legislation. We will also set up a national forum for people with learning disabilities and enable them to benefit from the improvement and expansion of community equipment services now under way.

- A person-centred approach will be essential to deliver real change in the lives of people with learning disabilities. Person-centred planning provides a single, multi-agency mechanism for achieving this. The Government will issue new guidance on person-centred planning, and provide resources for implementation through the Learning Disability Development Fund.

Supporting Carers

- Caring for a family member with a learning disability is a lifelong commitment. Our objective is to increase the help and support carers receive from all local agencies in order to fulfil their family and caring roles effectively.

- To help carers, we are providing **£750,000 over the next three years to fund the development of a national learning disability information centre and helpline in partnership with Mencap**. We will implement the Carers and Disabled Children Act 2000. Councils will be encouraged to identify carers aged over 70 and those from minority ethnic communities. We will also ensure that carers and their organisations are represented on the Learning Disability Task Force.

- Carers will benefit from our package of extra help worth more than £500 million over 3 years, which the Government announced in the autumn of 2000. In April 2001, the carer premium in the income-related benefits will rise to £24.40 a week, and the Invalid Care Allowance (ICA) earnings limit will rise to £72 a week. As soon as the legislative programme allows, people aged 65 and over will be able to claim ICA and entitlement to ICA will continue for up to 8 weeks after the death of the disabled person, to allow carers time to adjust.

Improving Health For People With Learning Disabilities

- Many people with learning disabilities have greater health needs than the rest of the population. They are more likely to experience mental illness and are more prone to chronic health problems, epilepsy, and physical and sensory disabilities. The Government's objective is to enable people with learning disabilities to have access to a health service designed around their individual needs, with fast and convenient care delivered to a consistently high standard and with additional support where necessary.

- We will ensure that people with learning disabilities, including those from minority ethnic communities, have **the same right of access to mainstream health services** as the rest of the population. The NHS will promote equality for people with learning disabilities from minority ethnic communities in accordance with its new general duty in the Race Relations (Amendment) Act 2000, which comes into force on 2 April 2001. **Health facilitators** will be appointed from each local community learning disability team to support people with learning disabilities in getting the health care they need. We will ensure that all people with learning disabilities are **registered with a GP** and have their own **Health Action Plan**. There will be a new role for specialist learning disability services, focusing on making best use of their expertise.

Housing, Fulfilling Lives, and Employment

- **Housing**. People with learning disabilities and their families currently have few options about where they live. Our objective is to enable people with learning disabilities and their families to have greater choice and control over where and how they live. We are legislating to improve provision of advice and information by housing authorities, and will be issuing joint DH/DETR guidance on housing care and support options. We will complete the reprovision of the remaining long-stay hospitals to enable people still living there to move to more appropriate accommodation in the community by 2004.

- **Fulfilling Lives**. Our objective is to enable people with learning disabilities to lead full and purposeful lives in their communities and develop a range of activities including leisure interests, friendships and relationships. To achieve this, we will take forward a 5 year programme to modernise local councils' day services. The Learning and Skills Council will ensure equal access to education. We will outlaw discrimination against people with learning disabilities on public transport. Services for parents with a learning disability will be improved. Department of Social Security staff will receive disability awareness training to help them work with people with learning disabilities.

- **Employment**. Very few people with learning disabilities – probably less than 10% – have jobs. Our objective is to enable more people with learning disabilities to participate in all forms of employment, wherever possible in paid work, and to make a valued contribution to the world of work. We will develop **new targets for increasing numbers of people with learning disabilities in work** and ensure that the Workstep programme meets the needs of people with learning disabilities. There will be a study of the links between supported employment and day services. The Department of Social Security will ensure careful assessment of entitlement to Disability Living Allowance. Job Brokers under the New Deal for Disabled People will have the skills needed to work with people with learning disabilities.

Quality Services

- The Government is committed to raising standards and improving the quality of services for people with learning disabilities. Good quality services that promote independence, choice and inclusion will lead to good outcomes for people with learning disabilities. We will look to the Social Care Institute of Excellence to be a leading source of expertise. Local quality assurance frameworks for learning disability will be in place by April 2002. We will issue guidance on user surveys and on physical intervention. We are taking action to assist vulnerable or intimidated witnesses to give evidence in Court and so improve their access to justice.

- At present, most of the learning disability workforce is unqualified. The Government wants to see an appropriately trained and qualified workforce. Health and social care workforce strategies will provide new opportunities for learning disability staff. We will also introduce the **Learning Disability Awards Framework** from April 2001 which will provide a new route to qualification for care staff. We will also support a range of leadership initiatives through the Learning Disability Development Fund.

- Good quality services will provide the right care for people with additional or complex needs. This includes people with severe and profound disabilities, people with learning disabilities and epilepsy, those with learning disabilities and autism, people with challenging behaviour and older people with learning disabilities.

Delivering Change

Partnership Working

- Effective partnership working by all agencies is the key to achieving social inclusion for people with learning disabilities. To promote stronger local partnerships, we will build on existing joint planning structures to establish Learning Disability Partnership Boards within the framework of Local Strategic Partnerships by October 2001. Partnership Boards will be responsible for agreeing plans for the use of the Health Act flexibilities.

Making Change Happen

- Delivering these ambitious plans will take time and requires a long-term implementation programme. At national level, we will be investing new resources in 2001/02 to support implementation. We will:

- Set up a **Learning Disability Task Force** to advise the Government on implementation;

- Establish an **Implementation Support Team** to promote change at regional and local level;

- Fund a £2 million learning disability research initiative *People with Learning disabilities: Services, Inclusion and Partnership* from 2001/02;

- At a local level, Learning Disability Partnership Boards will have lead responsibility for ensuring implementation. They will need to develop local action plans by 31 January 2002 to supplement their learning disability Joint Investment Plans;

- The Social Services Inspectorate will carry out a national inspection of learning disability services in 2001/02.

PREFACE

1   *Valuing People: A New Strategy for Learning Disability for the 21st Century* sets out the Government's proposals for improving the lives of people with learning disabilities and their families and carers, based on recognition of their rights as citizens, social inclusion in local communities, choice in their daily lives and real opportunities to be independent.

2   Developing these proposals involved extensive consultation over more than a year with key interests in the learning disability field:

- The Department of Health's national Learning Disability Advisory Group and the Service Users Advisory Group were consulted on emerging ideas;

- Six working groups bringing together people with learning disabilities, carers[2], local authority, NHS, and voluntary sector representatives, and researchers, as well as the key government departments, advised us on services for children, carers, health services, supporting independence, workforce training and planning, and building partnerships;

- Seven workshops across the country attended by almost 1,000 people, including people with learning disabilities and carers;

- Seminars on particular themes such as parents with learning disabilities, and consultation with disabled children were held to produce ideas for improving services;

- Other contributions came through our dedicated website (www.doh.gov.uk/learningdisabilities).

3   People with learning disabilities played an important part in the consultation process. Their contribution has been of central importance.

---

1   All the quotes are from people with learning disabilities came from the consultation process.
2   The carers who helped us develop the new strategy prefer to describe themselves as 'family carer' because this emphasises the family relationship. The Department of Health uses the term 'carer' to describe people who are not paid for caring and 'care worker' for people who are paid to work as carers.

4   Clear messages emerged from this consultation:

- **Children with learning disabilities** want to be treated like other children, not always seen as "special", and to be included in ordinary activities;

- **Parents of disabled children** want better advice and information and an integrated approach from services. Their expectations are often disappointed;

- **People with learning disabilities** often feel excluded and unheard. They want to be fully part of our society, not marginalised or forgotten. They told us advocacy and direct payments were key to helping them gain greater independence and control;

- **People with severe learning disabilities and complex needs** are more likely to receive poor quality services;

- **Carers** feel strongly that they have a lifelong responsibility for their sons or daughters. They want to be treated as full partners by public agencies. They need better information and support.

Our new strategy shows how the Government will respond to these concerns.

5   We also commissioned three reports which are being published to accompany *Valuing People*:

- **Nothing about Us Without Us: the report from the Service Users Advisory Group:** For the first time, people with learning disabilities have played a direct part in formulating Government policy. The members of the Service Users Advisory Group conducted a series of visits to local groups of learning disabled people. Listening to what people with learning disabilities had to tell us about their lives has helped us understand the need for change.

- **Family Matters, Counting Families In:** The report from the family carers working group offers valuable insights into the reality of service provision based on lifelong experience of caring for someone with a learning disability.

- **Learning Difficulties and Ethnicity,**[3] by the Centre for Research in Primary Care, University of Leeds. People with learning disabilities from minority ethnic communities and their families are too often overlooked. Meeting their needs is essential to providing a good service.

---

3   The authors use the term 'learning difficulties' as this was the preferred term among user organisations and disability writers.

PART ONE

WHERE WE ARE NOW

CHAPTER 1

PROBLEMS AND CHALLENGES

1.1 People with learning disabilities are amongst the most socially excluded and vulnerable groups in Britain today. Very few have jobs, live in their own homes or have real choice over who cares for them. Many have few friends outside their families and those paid to care for them. Their voices are rarely heard in public. This needs to change.

'It's about time we had something for ourselves'
(Gary)

1.2 It is thirty years since the last White Paper on learning disability services *Better Services for the Mentally Handicapped*, was published. Our new agenda needs to be based on social inclusion, civil rights, choice and independence. People with learning disabilities have the right to be full members of the society in which they live, to choose where they live and what they do, and to be as independent as they wish to be.

1.3 Achieving this aim requires all parts of Government to work in partnership. Social care, health, education, employment, housing, leisure and social security all have a part to play, with local councils taking a lead to ensure that partnership becomes a reality at local level.

What is Learning Disability?

1.4 *Valuing People* is based on the premise that people with learning disabilities are people first. We focus throughout on what people can do, with support where necessary, rather than on what they cannot do.

1.5 Learning disability includes the presence of:

- A significantly reduced ability to understand new or complex information, to learn new skills (impaired intelligence), with;

- A reduced ability to cope independently (impaired social functioning);

- which started before adulthood, with a lasting effect on development.

1.6 This definition encompasses people with a broad range of disabilities. The presence of a low intelligence quotient, for example an IQ below 70, is not, of itself, a sufficient reason for deciding whether an individual should be provided with additional health and social care support. An assessment of social functioning and communication skills should also be taken into account when determining need. Many people with learning disabilities also have physical and/or sensory impairments. The definition covers adults with autism who also have learning disabilities, but not those with a higher level autistic spectrum disorder who may be of average or even above average intelligence – such as some people with Asperger's Syndrome. We consider the additional needs of people with learning disability and autism in more detail in Chapter 8.

1.7 'Learning disability' does not include all those who have a 'learning difficulty' which is more broadly defined in education legislation.

How many people have learning disabilities?

1.8 Producing precise information on the number of people with learning disabilities[4] in the population is difficult. In the case of people with severe and profound learning disabilities, we estimate there are about 210,000: around 65,000 children and young people, 120,000 adults of working age and 25,000 older people. In the case of people with mild/moderate learning disabilities, lower estimates suggest a prevalence rate of around 25 per 1000 population- some 1.2 million people in England.

Figure 1 – People with learning disabilities, 1999

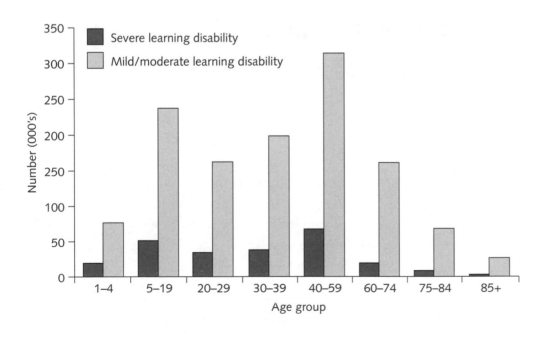

---

4 People with severe learning disabilities are those who need significant help with daily living. People with mild/moderate learning disabilities will usually be able to live independently with support.

1.9 Prevalence of severe and profound learning disability is fairly uniformly distributed across the country and across socio-economic groups. Mild to moderate learning disability, however, has a link to poverty and rates are higher in deprived and urban areas. The number of people with severe and profound learning disabilities in some areas is affected by past funding and placement practices, especially the presence of old long-stay patients and people placed outside their original area of residence by funding authorities.

Future Numbers

1.10 Evidence suggests that the number of people with severe learning disabilities may increase by around 1% per annum for the next 15 years as a result of:

- increased life expectancy, especially among people with Down's syndrome;

- growing numbers of children and young people with complex and multiple disabilities who now survive into adulthood;

- a sharp rise in the reported numbers of school age children with autistic spectrum disorders, some of whom will have learning disabilities;

- greater prevalence among some minority ethnic populations of South Asian origin.

Developments Since 1971

1.11 Until the 1950s, it was generally accepted that people with learning disabilities could enjoy a better quality of life living with other disabled people in segregated institutions rather than in the community with their families. The terms "mental deficiency" and "mental sub-normality" reflected the underlying attitudes of the day. Until 1959 those who lived in long-stay institutions were detained under the Mental Deficiency Act. By the end of the 1960s it became clear that the quality of care in long-stay hospitals was often extremely poor. Parental pressure became an important influence in the drive for change. The 1970 Education Act ensured that education should be provided for all children, no matter how severe their disability.

1.12 The 1971 White Paper *Better Services for the Mentally Handicapped* paved the way for change. It set an agenda for the next two decades which focused on reducing the number of places in hospitals and increasing provision in the community. It committed the

Government to helping people with learning disabilities to live "as normal a life" as possible, without unnecessary segregation from the community. It emphasised the importance of close collaboration between health, social services and other local agencies.

1.13 In 1971 the Government recognised that achieving change would require "sustained action over many years", and the White Paper set national targets (for England and Wales) for development of services which would take 15 to 20 years to achieve. These included reducing the number of long-stay hospital places for adults from 52,000 to 27,000 and increasing the number of residential care places in the community from 4,000 to nearly 30,000. Day places in the community needed to increase by nearly 50,000. Long-stay hospital places for children were to reduce from 7,400 to 6,400.

1.14 Many of the aims of the 1971 White Paper have been achieved. Very few large institutions remain and there are no children in long-stay hospitals. Services in the community have expanded and developed, and more people with learning disabilities are in work. There are active self-advocacy and citizen advocacy movements and the voices of people with learning disabilities are heard more clearly.

1971 White Paper	Services in 2000
In 1969, there were 58,850 patients (adults and children) in NHS hospitals or units	Nearly 10,000 places in NHS facilities: 1,570 NHS long-stay places 1,550 NHS specialist places 1,520 NHS campus places 5,100 places in residential accommodation managed by the NHS
4,900 places in residential care homes	53,400 places in residential care
24,500 places in Adult Training Centres	Estimated 84,000 adults receiving community based services (day care, home help, meals etc), of whom 49,600 are in receipt of social services day services 6,630 patients using NHS day care facilities

1.14 But more needs to be done. Too many people with learning disabilities and their families still lead lives apart, with limited opportunities and poor life chances. To maintain the momentum of change we now need to open up mainstream services, not create further separate specialist services. People with learning disabilities should have the same opportunities as other people to lead full and active lives and should receive the support needed to make this possible. The Government's agenda for reforming health and social care, modernising local government, promoting inclusive education and lifelong learning and Welfare to Work all offer major opportunities for improving the lives of people with learning disabilities. This can be done without losing the specialist expertise that currently exists.

Services and Expenditure

1.15 Many people with learning disabilities need additional support and services throughout their lives. This means that they have a longer and more intense involvement with public services than the vast majority of citizens. Services must provide them with safe, good quality care that delivers value for money.

1.16 Large amounts of public money are spent on learning disability services. Provisional health and social services expenditure on adults alone in 1999/2000 was over £3 billion: £1.4 billion on health and £1.6 billion on social services. In addition, about £308 million was spent by social services and £177 million by health on supporting disabled children, though not all of them have learning disabilities.

Figure 2 – Health and Local Authority Expenditure on Learning Disability

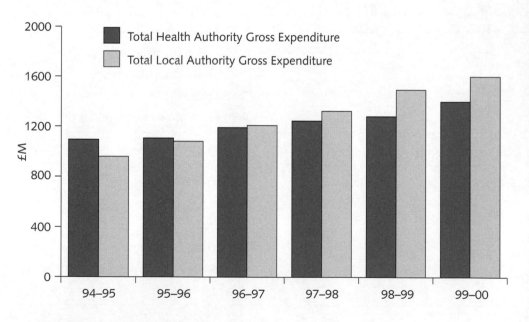

The figures for 1999/2000 are provisional.

1.17 The expansion of and improvement in some services has undoubtedly led to better outcomes for many people with learning disabilities. However, this does not mean services fully meet their needs. Research has consistently shown: variable quality of community based services; concerns about shortfalls of provision in particular services; and varying degrees of commitment to learning disability services by local authorities and health authorities.

Problems Facing Learning Disability Services

Social Exclusion

1.18 Despite the efforts of some highly committed staff, public services have failed to make consistent progress in overcoming the social exclusion of people with learning disabilities. These are some of the issues to be addressed:

Families with disabled children have higher costs as a result of the child's disability coupled with diminished employment prospects. Their housing needs may not be adequately met. There is little evidence of a flexible and co-ordinated approach to support by health, education and social services, and there is significant unmet need for short breaks.

Young disabled people at the point of transition to adult life often leave school without a clear route towards a fulfilling and productive adult life.

Carers can feel undervalued by public services, lacking the right information and enough support to meet their lifelong caring responsibilities.

Choice and Control. Many people with learning disabilities have little choice or control in their lives. Recent research shows only 6% of people with learning disabilities having control over who they lived with and 1% over choice of carer. Advocacy services are patchy and inconsistent. Direct payments have been slow to take off for people with learning disabilities.

Health Care. The substantial health care needs of people with learning disabilities too often go unmet. They can experience avoidable illness and die prematurely.

Housing can be the key to achieving social inclusion, but the number supported to live independently in the community, for example, remains small. Many have no real choice and receive little advice about possible housing options.

Day services frequently fail to provide sufficiently flexible and individual support. Some large day centres offer little more than warehousing and do not help people with learning disabilities undertake a wider range of individually tailored activities.

Social Isolation remains a problem for too many people with learning disabilities. A recent study[5] found that only 30% had a friend who was not either learning disabled, or part of their family or paid to care for them.

Employment is a major aspiration for people with learning disabilities, but less than 10% nationally are in work, so most people remain heavily dependent on social security benefits.

The needs of people with learning disabilities from minority ethnic communities are too often overlooked. Key findings from the study by the Centre for Research in Primary Care at the University of Leeds published alongside *Valuing People* included:

- prevalence of learning disability in some South Asian communities can be up to three times greater than in the general population;

- diagnosis is often made at a later age than for the population as a whole and parents receive less information about their child's condition and the support available;

- social exclusion is made more severe by language barriers and racism, and negative stereotypes and attitudes contribute to disadvantage;

- carers who do not speak English receive less information about their support role and experience high levels of stress; and

- agencies often underestimate people's attachments to cultural traditions and religious beliefs.

Inconsistency in Service Provision

1.19 The national statistics on learning disability conceal great variation across the country in terms of availability and coverage of services, as well as quality. Findings from three recent Department of Health studies of local authorities and their comparable health authorities – *Facing The Facts,*[6] *The London Learning Disability Strategic Framework* and a survey of 24 local authorities carried out during the development of the new strategy – show we are far from achieving consistency and equity for people with learning disabilities and their families.

---

5   The Quality and Costs of Residential Supports for People with Learning Disabilities, Summary & Implications (Hester Adrian Research Centre, University of Manchester, 1999).

6   Facing the Facts: Services for People with Learning Disabilities – A Policy Impact Study of Social Care and Health Services (Department of Health 1999).

1.20 The main variations in social services and the NHS include:

- **Expenditure:** In London, social services expenditure per 10,000 population ranges from under £200,000 to £500,000. Health spend per 10,000 population ranges from under £100,000 to £450,000;

- **Day Services:** attendance at day centres ranges from 3 to 198 per 10,000 population, with higher figures generally associated with traditional day centres. Cost per attendance ranged from £18 to £112. We also know that some 20,000 people with learning disabilities – often the most severely disabled or those with challenging behaviour – do not attend a day service;

- **Short Breaks:** *Facing the Facts* found that the number of bed nights paid for by local authorities per 10,000 population ranged from 25 in a unitary authority to 492 in a shire county. For the special survey the range was 1 to 406 per 10,000 population. The last national Social Services Inspectorate inspection[7] found that short breaks were generally in short supply; and

- **Accommodation:** across the country the number of adults receiving care in publicly funded accommodation ranges from 12.74 per 10,000 population aged 18–64 to 59.20. Few places offer real choice.

1.21 The Government is committed to tackling the postcode lottery revealed here. It will be one of the key challenges in implementing the new strategy.

Management of Services

1.22 Good management of learning disability services requires:

- **strong partnership working:** while learning disability has been at the forefront of making use of the flexibilities under the Health Act 1999, many areas have yet to achieve real partnership between health and social care. Joint commissioning has been slow to take off. Few areas have partnerships involving service users, their families and the wider range of agencies.

- **good planning to ensure that services are responsive:** Few places attempt to have the individual's aspirations, needs and views as the driving force for providing services.

---

7 Moving into the Mainstream: The Report of a National Inspection of Services for Adults with Learning Disabilities (Department of Health 1998)

- **a highly skilled workforce:** we know that levels of training and qualification in the learning disability workforce remain low and there are shortages of key professionals and care staff.

The Way Forward

1.23 There is no "quick fix" solution to these problems; tackling them requires radical change from all of us. We need to develop a new approach to delivering better life chances for people with learning disabilities. We can no longer tolerate services which leave people isolated and marginalised. Good quality public services should offer new opportunities for people with learning disabilities to lead full and productive lives as valued members of their local communities. Our proposals are intended to:

- tackle social exclusion and achieve better life chances;

- ensure value for money from the large public investment in learning disability services;

- reduce variation and promote consistency and equity of services across the country;

- promote effective partnership working at all levels to ensure a really person-centred approach to delivering quality services;

- drive up standards by encouraging an evidence-based approach to service provision and practice.

CHAPTER 2

THE NEW VISION

2.1 Improving the lives of people with learning disabilities requires commitment nationally and locally to strong principles, a firm value base and clear objectives for services. Each individual should have the support and opportunity to be the person he or she wants to be.

Key Principles: Rights, Independence, Choice, and Inclusion

2.2 There are four key principles at the heart of the Government's proposals in *Valuing People*:

Legal and Civil Rights: The Government is committed to enforceable civil rights for disabled people in order to eradicate discrimination in society. People with learning disabilities have the right to a decent education, to grow up to vote, to marry and have a family, and to express their opinions, with help and support to do so where necessary. The Government is committed to providing comprehensive guidance for electoral administrators on helping disabled people, including those with learning disabilities, through the whole electoral process – from registering to vote until polling day itself.

All public services will treat people with learning disabilities as individuals with respect for their dignity, and challenge discrimination on all grounds including disability. People with learning disabilities will also receive the full protection of the law when necessary.

Independence: Promoting independence is a key aim for the Government's modernisation agenda. Nowhere is it of greater importance than for people with learning disabilities. While people's individual needs will differ, the starting presumption should be one of independence, rather than dependence, with public services providing the support needed to maximise this. Independence in this context does not mean doing everything unaided.

"People with learning disabilities are citizens too"

"All this can be done ... by believing that people with learning disabilities can move on and be independent"

"People with learning disabilities have been saying for a long time that we can speak up for ourselves"

"People with learning disabilities can live just as good a life"

Choice: Like other people, people with learning disabilities want a real say in where they live, what work they should do and who looks after them. But for too many people with learning disabilities, these are currently unattainable goals. We believe that everyone should be able to make choices. This includes people with severe and profound disabilities who, with the right help and support, can make important choices and express preferences about their day to day lives.

Inclusion: Being part of the mainstream is something most of us take for granted. We go to work, look after our families, visit our GP, use transport, go to the swimming pool or cinema. Inclusion means enabling people with learning disabilities to do those ordinary things, make use of mainstream services and be fully included in the local community.

Our Values

2.3 Our new proposals reflect these four key principles and we set out below how they can be realised at both national and local level. They are grounded in the legislation that confers rights on all citizens including people with learning disabilities:

- the Human Rights Act 1998;

- the Disability Discrimination Act 1995;

- the Race Relations Act 1976;

- the Race Relations (Amendment) Act 2000;

- the Sex Discrimination Act 1975; and

- the UN Convention on the Rights of the Child, which was adopted in the UK in January 1992.

2.4 The Disability Rights Commission established in April 2000 has a vital role to play in enabling all disabled people, including those with learning disabilities, to gain full access to their legal rights. It will ensure that the needs and views of people with learning disabilities are integral to all the Commission's work.

2.5 People who are vulnerable to exploitation have to be protected in law. The position of those who are vulnerable to sexual abuse and exploitation is considered in the report of the Sex Offences Review *Setting the Boundaries*. This includes discussion on the capacity to consent for very vulnerable people. That report recommends a new offence of a breach of a relationship of care which would cover sexual relationships between, for example, doctors and their patients, or between designated care providers and people receiving certain care services in the community.

Government Objectives for Learning Disability Services

2.6 If public services are to continue to improve we need both to set a clear direction and create clear objectives. The new Government objectives developed from our consultation process set out below provide this direction for all agencies working with people with learning disabilities. They are an essential first step in tackling unacceptable variation and promoting greater consistency and equity in services.

2.7 Our objectives reflect the partnership approach which is central to Valuing People and clarify the Government's expectations of all local agencies providing help to people with learning disabilities and their carers: social services, health, education, employment, housing, the Benefits Agency, transport and leisure services. Local voluntary groups and independent service providers also need to be part of the partnership. This approach is in line with the Government's principles for partnership working enshrined in the Local Strategic Partnerships now being introduced to co-ordinate implementation of local community strategies and the Government's strategy for neighbourhood renewal. Our partnership proposals set out in Chapter 9 will fit within the umbrella provided by Local Strategic Partnerships.

2.8 There are two categories of Government objectives for people with learning disabilities: the first deal with outcomes for people and the second concern systems needed in order to deliver better outcomes. We support the objectives with more detailed sub-objectives, which will be monitored through new performance indicators. Annex A contains the complete list.

2.9 These objectives will provide the focus for local action to implement our proposals. We will require local agencies to build on the Joint Investment Plans which are already expected to be in place for April 2001 in order to develop local action plans. Chapter 10 looks in further detail at the role and contents of these plans, along with arrangements for monitoring the implementation of the White Paper as a whole.

Objective 1: Maximising Opportunities for Disabled Children
To ensure that disabled children gain maximum life chance benefits from educational opportunities, health care and social care, while living with their families or in other appropriate settings in the community where their assessed needs are adequately met and reviewed.

Objective 2: Transition into Adult Life
As young people with learning disabilities move into adulthood, to ensure continuity of care and support for the young person and their family and to provide equality of opportunity in order to enable as many disabled young people as possible to participate in education, training or employment.

Objective 3: Enabling People To Have More Control Over Their Own Lives
To enable people with learning disabilities to have as much choice and control as possible over their lives through advocacy and a person-centred approach to planning the services they need

Objective 4: Supporting Carers
To increase the help and support carers receive from all local agencies in order to fulfil their family and caring roles effectively.

Objective 5: Good Health
To enable people with learning disabilities to access a health service designed around their individual needs, with fast and convenient care delivered to a consistently high standard, and with additional support where necessary.

Objective 6: Housing
To enable people with learning disabilities and their families to have greater choice and control over where, and how they live.

Objective 7: Fulfilling Lives
To enable people with learning disabilities to lead full and purposeful lives in their communities and to develop a range of friendships, activities and relationships.

Objective 8: Moving into Employment
To enable more people with learning disabilities to participate in all forms of employment, wherever possible in paid work and to make a valued contribution to the world of work.

Objective 9: Quality
To ensure that all agencies commission and provide high quality, evidence based and continuously improving services which promote both good outcomes and best value.

Objective 10. Workforce Training and Planning
To ensure that social and health care staff working with people with learning disabilities are appropriately skilled, trained and qualified, and to promote a better understanding of the needs of people with learning disabilities amongst the wider workforce.

Objective 11: Partnership Working
To promote holistic services for people with learning disabilities through effective partnership working between all relevant local agencies in the commissioning and delivery of services.

Action for Change

2.9   *Valuing People* sets out a major programme to improve life chances
for people with learning disabilities. The Government will:

- Set out a new vision for services for disabled children and their
families, to be delivered through an integrated approach by
health, education and social care. Disabled children will be fully
included as an integral part of the Government's major reform
agenda for all children and families. The Quality Protects
programme targets £60 million over the next three years on
improving support for disabled children and their families;

- Enable disabled young people to have equal opportunities
for moving into adult life, with new support from the
Connexions Service;

- Give people with learning disabilities more choice and control
by developing advocacy, extending direct payments and
introducing a national framework for promoting a person-
centred approach to planning. The Government is investing
£1.3 million per annum for the next three years in establishing
a National Citizen Advocacy Network and promoting self-
advocacy, both in partnership with the voluntary sector;

- Provide £750,000 over the next three years to establish a
National Learning Disability Information Centre and Helpline
in partnership with Mencap;

- Enable all people with learning disabilities to have access to
a health facilitator and to have a Health Action Plan;

- Complete the reprovision of the remaining long-stay hospitals
to enable everyone still living there to move to more
appropriate accommodation by April 2004;

- Take forward a five year programme for modernising day
services to provide more individualised support, with clear
targets and bridging finance;

- Set a new Government target for increasing employment for
people with learning disabilities, backed by the development
of local employment strategies;

- Introduce the new Learning Disability Awards Framework in
April 2001 to provide a new route to qualification for care
workers in the learning disability field; and

- Strengthen partnership working by giving local councils lead responsibility for establishing new Learning Disability Partnership Boards. These will build on existing partnership structures to bring together public, voluntary and independent agencies and the wider community within the overall framework of Local Strategic Partnerships. Partnership Boards will be responsible for implementation of the White Paper and will need to submit updated Joint Investment Plans (JIPs) setting out plans for local action to the Department of Health by 31 January 2002.

2.10 Making these changes happen requires a long-term implementation programme over at least the next five years. The Government will provide a strong national lead and will:

- Introduce a new Learning Disability Development Fund of up to £50 million from April 2002: up to £30 million per annum revenue and £20 million capital. The revenue element of the Fund will be created from NHS old long-stay funding as it is released overtime. Resources from the Fund may only be used where they are deployed as part of pooled budgets under the Health Act flexibilities enabling them to be targeted on supporting our key proposals;

- Establish a Learning Disability Task Force, bringing together a wide range of expertise including people with learning disabilities and carers;

- Set up a national Implementation Support Team; and

- Introduce a new Implementation Support Fund of £2.3 million a year for the next 3 years.

2.11 Chapters 3 to 8 set out the problems and challenges facing people with learning disabilities, their families, their carers and agencies providing services, describe what is currently being done and list the key actions to be taken to help address the problems.

PART TWO:

BETTER LIFE CHANCES FOR

PEOPLE WITH LEARNING

DISABILITIES

CHAPTER 3

DISABLED CHILDREN AND YOUNG PEOPLE

Government Objective: To ensure that disabled children gain maximum life chance benefits from educational opportunities, health care and social care, while living with their families or in other appropriate settings in the community where their assessed needs are adequately met and reviewed.

3.1　This chapter sets out the Government's proposals for maximising opportunities for disabled children and supporting young people's transition into adult life. It focuses in particular on the needs of learning disabled children and their families, but does so within a framework which applies equally to all disabled children. Many disabled children have more than one impairment and a majority have a learning disability. There are an estimated 1.7 million pupils in schools with special educational needs, of whom some 250,000 have statements of special educational need. Most of those children with statements will also be defined as disabled. We will build on existing health, social services and education programmes to develop an integrated approach to supporting disabled children. Children and their families want services that are not only efficient and effective, but also joined up and responsive. We propose to set new Government objectives and sub-objectives to be applied from April 2002. (See Annex A).

Problems and Challenges

3.2　Society creates many problems and poses many challenges for disabled children and their families. Despite these, many families are very successful in providing a good start in life for their disabled children. There is a compelling body of evidence from research and inspection reports that disabled children and their families face many barriers to full participation in society:

- too little family support, help in the home and too few short breaks especially for more severely disabled children;

- too often living in poverty;

- lack of key workers leading to poorly co-ordinated inter-agency support;

- frequent delay in diagnosis and identification of the child's impairments;

- lack of good information about what help is available;

- limited expectation of children's educational achievements;

- some children live in residential placements, which can increase isolation from home and family and increase vulnerability to abuse;

- too few opportunities to participate in sport, culture and leisure activities;

- inequalities in access and quality of NHS services;

- minority ethnic families experience these barriers disproportionately;

- lack of opportunities for disabled young people moving into adulthood.

3.3   Three main messages have come out of consultation with disabled children:

- treat us more like our brothers and sisters,

- we want to do the things other children do, not always 'something special', and

- give us a chance to be independent, get a job and have a home.

3.4   Research findings show parents of disabled children would like:

- key workers to help co-ordinate services;

- early identification of impairments and early intervention;

- simple accessible information about available services;

- greater access to family support, short breaks and support.

What more needs to be done

KEY ACTIONS – DISABLED CHILDREN

- New priority in Quality Protects programme: £60m of children's services grant earmarked for more support for families of disabled children from 2001/2 to 2003/4, resulting in more home based help and more access to key workers.

- Major Government programme to improve educational outcomes for children with special needs, based on collaborative working across health, education and social services.

- £220 million from 2001 to 2004 to improve the accessibility of mainstream schools for disabled children.

- A new duty on all LEAs to provide parent partnership services for families of children with SEN, supported by £18m Standards Fund grant in 2001/02.

- Joint DH/DFEE work on position of children in residential placements.

- Additional family support through statutory and voluntary sectors including co-ordinated health and social care packages to an additional 6,000 severely disabled children by 2002.

- From April 2001 the introduction of direct payments to give parents and disabled 16- and 17-year-olds greater choice in how they receive services.

- New National Information Centre for families of disabled children to be launched in 2001 by Contact a Family. Government funding of £500,000 per annum.

- Action to enable more disabled children to use sport, culture and leisure activities.

- £4m ringfenced in National Childcare Strategy for children with disabilities and SEN, enabling more staff to be employed to support disabled children.

- A multi-agency working party to develop practical guidance for professionals involved in identifying the special needs of children in the 0–2 age bracket.

- Early support and intervention to tackle the social exclusion of disabled children through cross Government programmes (Sure Start, The Children's Fund and Connexions).

- Improved social security benefits for families with disabled children, helping reduce child poverty.

- A new National Service Framework for children to reduce health inequalities and ensure that all children have fair access to and high standards of health care.

- Development of integrated services for children and young people with severe disabilities and complex needs a priority for use of the capital element of the Learning Disability Development Fund.

- New transition arrangements, through the Connexions Service, to improve opportunities for disabled young people to take part in education, training or employment.

Quality Protects Programme

3.5   The Quality Protects programme set up to improve children's social services will:

- increase provision of a wider range of flexible support services for families of disabled children including short breaks;

- help integrate disabled children into mainstream leisure and out of school services;

- provide more and better information for families and increase the availability of key workers and other measures to improve co-ordination.

3.6   From April 2001 disabled children will be included in the priority areas for the grant. £60m has been earmarked for services for disabled children and their families – £15 million in 2001/2002 and 2002/2003 and £30 million in 2003/2004.

Family Support

3.7   The Government has set a target for an additional 6,000 severely disabled children by 2002 to receive support by a co-ordinated care package from health and social services.

3.8   The Government is increasing funding to the Family Fund Trust which provides grants to help reduce the stress on families with severely disabled children, including grants to pay for holidays, washing machines and other services. In 2000/2001, the Government contributed funding of £25.4 million. This funding will be increased by £1m in 2001/02, £2m in 2002/03 and £3m in 2003/4.

The Cheviots Centre

The Cheviots Centre in Enfield provides a range of services to children who have severe learning disabilities, very challenging behaviour problems and life limiting conditions. They provide a range of core services to give families the support they need to be able to look after their disabled child at home. The Centre provides a service which is seamless, fast and responsive and includes: holiday play schemes; home care support; a counselling service and a range of activity groups which runs 7 days a week.

3.9 The Government will continue to support the Diana Children's Community Nursing Teams. These teams work in partnership with other local agencies and provide physical, social and emotional support to children with life limiting disorders in their own homes as an alternative to hospital-based care.

3.10 From April 2001 through the SEN Programme of Action, the Government will provide local education authorities with £18m to support the development of parent partnership services, and will invest a further £2m to pilot arrangements for independent parental supporters in the expectation that these will be available in all areas from 2002/03.

3.11 The implementation of the Carers and Disabled Children Act 2000 will allow direct payments to be made from April 2001 to parents of disabled children, giving greater choice and flexibility in how they receive services.

3.12 Families need to be able to make informed choices about the services and support they need for their children and for themselves. From 2001, the Government is funding the charity Contact a Family by £500,000 per annum for three years, to set up a new National Information Centre for families with disabled children. This will include a national telephone help and advice line for disabled children and parents.

Play, Leisure, Culture and Sport

3.13 Disabled children want support to do the things their peers do, such as going swimming or to a youth club. Participation in play and sporting activities can help build self-esteem and social skills. The Government is taking action by: increasing through the Quality Protects programme the numbers of disabled children involved in leisure and play activities; supporting 13% of New Opportunities Fund places going to children with special needs; ensuring that all children in Sure Start areas will have access to good quality play opportunities, including one to one support and adapted toys and equipment.

Education Services

SEN PROGRAMME OF ACTION

3.14 Education, as a key service for children, must be characterised by its inclusiveness and its high expectations for all children, including those children with special educational needs, and those who are disabled. The Government's aim is to encourage disabled children

The Markfield Project

'To make the **best** playscheme ever we all promise:

To be nice and kind. To be treated with respect. To not swear or spit. Not to shout. To call people by their names and not 'oi'. Not to play with peoples wheelchairs. To have FREEDOM to play. A lot of excitement and fun. To be included. TO play FUN games. To not kick, hit or bully each other. To play with everyone and make new friends. To listen and be listened to. To have a GOOD time! TO be helped when needed. To go on trips, have adventures and learn new things.'

Promised by the children and staff on the summer playscheme 2000

to reach their full potential. The SEN Programme of Action is committed to:

i)   improving early identification and early intervention;

ii) supporting parents and carers;

iii) improving the SEN framework;

iv) developing a more inclusive education system;

v)   developing knowledge and skills;

vi) working in partnership.

3.15 Through the programme the Government has pledged additional resources to improve the education of children with disabilities. From April 2001 £220m has been allocated, over three years, through the Schools Access Initiative, to improve the accessibility of mainstream schools. Further, for 2001–02, £82m in the Standards Fund is earmarked to improve provision for children with special educational needs.

3.16 The Government's Special Educational Needs and Disability Bill will:

- strengthen the right of children with SEN to be educated in mainstream schools;

- require LEAs to provide parents of children with SEN with advice and information, and a means of settling disputes with schools and LEAs;

- require schools to inform parents where they are making special educational provision for their child and allow schools to request a statutory assessment of a pupil's SEN;

- place duties to increase physical accessibility to school premises and to not treat disabled children less favourably compared to non disabled children;

- place new duties on schools and LEAs to make reasonable adjustments so disabled pupils are not placed at a substantial disadvantage to their non-disabled peers.

3.17 From 2002, the Government will use revised statistical arrangements to monitor the progress and attainment of children, including those with learning disabilities. All schools will set targets for the achievement of children working below age related expectations on the National Curriculum. Further, the Qualifications & Curriculum Authority will issue guidance to schools on target setting and assessment for children working below these age related expectations. This will help ensure higher expectations of and higher attainment by all children with special needs. The revised SEN Code of

Practice, together with practical guidance, will help schools better identify needs early and provide for those needs.

3.18 During 2001/02 the Department for Education and Employment and the Department and Health will build on this substantial programme by:

- developing guidance on good practice in early identification of SEN;

- issuing – alongside the revised SEN Code of Practice – practical guidance on involving disabled children in decisions about their education;

- working with the Disability Rights Commission on the production of a Code to help schools make reasonable adjustments to include disabled children fully in the life and curriculum of their school;

- helping schools share effective practice on the delivery of inclusive education;

- developing measures of attainment and personal and social development for children with SEN;

- ensure that health services, social care and family support services are provided as far as possible, in school, or in other ways which support children's education and the well being of families.

HEALTH CARE IN SCHOOLS

3.19 Many children with special needs in mainstream schools require considerable support from health and social services. Children should not be disadvantaged in terms of access to health care as a result of parents' choice of school. It is particularly important that a child's health treatment/therapy should be provided with minimum disruption to their education and, wherever possible, necessary health care support should be delivered through schools and in a way which supports families. The NHS Plan sets out the Government's commitment to provide 6,500 more NHS therapists and related professional staff by 2004, with 4,450 more training places. In the summer the Department of Health will issue guidance on implementation. This will encourage wider use of the Health Act flexibilities in order to develop more integrated partnership working.

3.20 The Department for Education and Employment is sponsoring a network of eleven SEN Regional Partnerships across England. These bring together groups of local education authorities, local health and social services plus the private and voluntary sectors. We will promote full collaboration in these partnerships and also across the Department of Health's regional task forces to ensure joined-up child centred services for disabled children.

3.21 *Saving Lives: Our Healthier Nation* set out a child-centred public health role for school nurses, working with individual children and young people, families, schools and communities to improve health and tackle inequality. Schools can have a tailored health plan agreed in partnership with the school nurse to address the health needs and education priorities of the school. School nurses will assess an individual child's health needs and initiate and develop programmes for children with medical or special education needs to maximise their learning potential, and to promote health and inclusion in school life.

Residential Placements

3.22 Some disabled children are placed in residential schools; others live in residential homes. Whilst many of these placements are highly valued by children and families, they may result in their isolation from normal childhood support. We do not know enough about these children. In 2001/02 the children in need census will help enable councils to identify how many disabled children are in residential homes. In 2001/02 the Department of Health and Department for Education and Employment will work together to find out more about the numbers, characteristics and outcomes relating to these children. We will develop arrangements which will create better linkages between children living in residential placements and their family, and ensure they are properly supported and protected by key agencies.

3.23 Disabled children living in residential placements are known to be particularly vulnerable to abuse. The Care Standards Act 2000 strengthens the safeguards for children living away from home. From April 2002, the new National Care Standards Commission will register children's homes (including those homes for disabled children currently registered as care homes) and inspect the welfare of children in all boarding schools and Further Education colleges with boarding provision. Separate standards will be introduced for residential special schools.

Early Years Developments

3.24 Early Years and Childcare Development Partnerships have a responsibility to ensure that all sectors of the community have equal access to childcare, regardless of their special educational needs or disability. From April 2001, £144.75 million will be available to support Partnerships' Plans. Included in this sum, is a ring-fenced amount of £ 4 million to provide childcare services for children with special educational needs or disabilities and other special groups. In addition Partnerships can, at their discretion, supplement this amount using their general childcare grant.

3.25 Current childcare tax credit rules do not support parents who use formal childcare in their own home. This poses a specific barrier to work for families with particular needs, such as those with disabled children who need home-based care. The Government announced in the 2001 Budget that it is to consider how these families might be helped, for example by extending the childcare tax credit to cover formal childcare in the home where it meets standards similar to those that will govern the regulation and accreditation of childminders.

3.26 The Early Excellence Centres programme is a test-bed for developing high quality integrated services for the early years. Participating centres offer integrated early education and childcare, family support and dissemination of good practice. There are now 35 centres with a key role in: supporting children and families with special educational needs; improving early identification of needs; promoting inclusion; enabling parents to cope. Evaluation of the pilot Early Excellence Centres found that they had increased the rates of inclusion in mainstream education for children identified as having SENs in early childhood and were cost effective.

3.27 The Government intends to establish a multi-agency working party, with representation from specialist organisations with an interest, to develop practical guidance for the range of professionals involved in identifying the special needs of children aged 0–2 and offering support to the children and their families. The guidance will provide examples of good practice and set out practical advice to help agencies enhance joint working.

Cross Government Programmes for Children and Young People

3.28 Disabled children will also benefit from three cross government programmes to help prevent vulnerable children and young people from becoming socially excluded:

- Sure Start partnerships help in identifying young children (0–4 year olds) with disabilities and ensuring the provision of early intervention and support. Targeted efforts are then made to ensure that identified children receive relevant support to help them enter successfully into early years education. The support by Sure Start includes support for families with special needs;

- The £450 million Children's Fund will help families of disabled children (primarily in the 5 to 13 age group) by support through multidisciplinary teams and local voluntary groups. Services might include support for parents of disabled children and mentoring schemes;

- The Connexions service will be available to help all young people (primarily 13–19-year-olds) make a successful transition from school to the world of work, training and further education. The Connexions Personal Advisers will have a key role in supporting disabled young people into adulthood.

Child Poverty

3.29 From April 2001, families with disabled children will benefit from the following:

- An increase in the disabled child premium in income related benefits by £7.40 per week on top of normal uprating. 80,000 families with disabled children will see a rise in this premium from £22.25 to £30 a week. This change will be mirrored by an increase from April 2001 of £7.40 a week over and above inflation of the disabled child tax credit in Working Families' Tax Credit and Disabled Person's Tax Credit;

- The Disabled Income Guarantee will be paid to families on low incomes with severely disabled children receiving the highest care component of Disability Living Allowance. Extra £11.05 a week for each eligible child;

- Severely disabled 3- and 4-year-olds will benefit from entitlement to the higher rate mobility component of Disability Living Allowance.

Health Services

ACCESS TO HEALTH CARE

3.30 Disabled children have exactly the same health care needs as other children in addition to any arising from their particular disabilities. The NHS provides a universal service for all based on clinical need and the Government is determined to ensure disabled children have the same access to services as other children. Discrimination on any grounds, including disability, has no place in the NHS. The Government has announced the development of a National Service Framework (NSF) for children. This will help us improve services for all children and families and ensure we reduce unacceptable variations in the standards of care and in access to care. As promised in the NHS Plan, the Government has also set targets for reducing inequalities in childhood mortality and is developing targets for reducing morbidity inequalities. From 2001 fair access to health care will be measured and managed through the NHS Performance Management Framework. We will also look further at how Patient Advocacy Liaison Groups (PALS) will help disabled children and their families.

DIAGNOSIS IN EARLY CHILDHOOD

3.31 The NHS programme of surveillance and screening of children enables children with disabilities to be identified at an early stage. We provide funding for the development of training packages and information aimed at all health professionals to improve their knowledge of disability and to enhance their skills in sharing this information sensitively with the child, their parents and other family members. Liaison nurses are increasingly being used to help families through the trauma of major medical surgical interventions and to provide ongoing support.

COMPLEX HEALTH NEEDS

3.32 The Government is concerned to support the increasing numbers of children with complex medical needs, some of whom are dependent on technology. We will take steps to establish the numbers and socio-economic characteristics of these children. Support for these families will be given through the Quality Protects programme and through the New Opportunity Fund providing grants for projects offering palliative care to children with life limiting illness and their families.

Rosehill and Littlemore Sure Start is developing work on early identification of special needs in children via a special needs support worker (a commissioned service from the LEA) who uses a particular form of intervention therapy. The Asian Families Liaison Worker (a commissioned service from Oxford City Council) found that identifying learning difficulties is a significant issue among children from Asian families. She is working with the special needs support worker via home visits, nursery and playgroup settings to offer individual and group support to adults and children in liaison with the locality health team.

3.33 In order to make further progress in improving services for children with complex needs and their families, we have made developing integrated health and social services facilities for such children and young people a priority area for the use of the capital element of the Learning Disability Development Fund.

CHILD AND ADOLESCENT MENTAL HEALTH SERVICES (CAMHS)

3.34 Children with physical or learning disabilities are more vulnerable to the full range of mental health disorders and the additional social, family and emotional stresses of everyday life. £50 million has already been allocated to improve child and adolescent mental health services over the period 1999 to 2001. The Government is committed to improving services for children and young people with mental health problems through the implementation of the NHS Plan. By May 2001, all health authorities and local councils must have an agreed joint CAMHS Development Strategy which sets out how local and national priorities are to be met, including 24-hour cover and outreach services and increasing early intervention and prevention programmes for children. Arrangements to provide CAMHS for learning disabled children will be included in all relevant planning arrangements for children.

TRANSITION INTO ADULT LIFE

Government Objective: As young people with learning disabilities move into adulthood, to ensure continuity of care and support for the young person and their family; and to provide equality of opportunity in order to enable as many disabled young people as possible to participate in education, training or employment.

Problems and Challenges

3.35 Disabled young people and their families often find the transition to adulthood both stressful and difficult. For many, there has been a lack of co-ordination between the relevant agencies and little involvement from the young person. Some young people are not transferred from children's to adult services with adequate health care plans, which results in their exclusion from adult services. This is likely to affect young people with severe learning disabilities and complex health needs in particular. Starting adult life should be a time of opportunity for young people. The Government wants to see more young people taking part in education and training, which will help them lead productive adult lives and find employment.

What more needs to be done

Making the Connexions Service work for Young People with Learning Disabilities

3.36 From April 2001, the new Connexions Service will be rolled out to provide all 13–19-year-olds with access to advice, guidance and support, through the creation of a network of personal advisers. These advisers will identify young people with learning disabilities; they must be invited to and attend annual reviews of all year 9 pupils with statements of SEN; and will work with the school and other relevant agencies to draw up the transition plans. Each Connexions Partnership must have sufficient Personal Advisers with the appropriate skills, experience and training to work with disabled young people. For young people leaving care the Children (Leaving Care) Act places a duty on councils to provide qualifying young people aged 16 and over in and leaving care with a personal adviser. There is such a significant overlap between the roles envisaged for the Act's advisers and Connexions advisers that the advisers provided by councils will also be well placed , with training, to act as Connexions advisers.

3.37 Connexions Partnerships will have responsibility for arranging with the local Learning and Skills Council and the Employment Service a review for the young person with learning disabilities in their 19th year, to agree arrangements for appropriate transition from the support provided by the Connexions Service, whilst ensuring continuity. Adult social services may need to be involved in some cases. Where young people are not ready to use the adult guidance services, Connexions Partnerships will continue to support them, with the aim of helping them make use of the adult systems and to reduce dependency on the Connexions Service. These arrangements can extend up to their 25th birthday.

Young People and Person-centred Planning

3.38 Chapter 4 sets out the Government's proposals for a person-centred approach to planning services for adults with learning disabilities. Local councils will take the lead in ensuring that local Learning Disability Partnership Boards responsible for planning and commissioning services for adults agree a framework for the

Connecting with Connexions – a Community Care Development Centre Project

Connexions pilot Personal Advisers (PAs) in Lewisham are exploring how to prepare young people with learning disabilities for the world of work. Two PAs appointed by London South Bank Careers to special schools are linking with two experienced supported employment agencies (Sabre and STATUS). The PAs are learning about supported employment and meeting job coaches and people with learning disabilities who have jobs. The outcome will be information about guidance and materials to help link Connexions with work options and how to support PAs to work with young people with learning disabilities.

development of person-centred planning. This will build on the assessment and planning for young people already undertaken by Connexions. The Government will issue further guidance on person-centred planning for adults with learning disabilities in 2001. Local agencies will be expected to have introduced person-centred planning for all young people moving from children's to adult's services by 2003.

3.39 There will also need to be effective links in place between children's and adults services in both health and social care. We will expect Learning Disability Partnership Boards to identify a member with lead responsibility for transition issues. Ensuring continuity in health care will be a key element of the new Health Action Plan for people with learning disabilities discussed in Chapter 6. For social care, the Director of Social Services will be required to ensure that good links are in place between children's and adult services for people with learning disabilities as part of his/her new responsibility for quality under the Social Care Quality Framework.

CHAPTER 4

MORE CHOICE AND CONTROL FOR PEOPLE WITH LEARNING DISABILITIES

Government Objective: To enable people with learning disabilities to have as much choice and control as possible over their lives through advocacy and a person-centred approach to planning the services and support they need.

The proposals in this chapter will be central to delivering the Government's four key principles. The rights of people with learning disabilities need to be promoted. They also need help in order to achieve greater choice, independence and inclusion in all aspects of their lives. Services should respond to the wider aspirations of people with learning disabilities and give them more choice and control.

Problems and Challenges

4.1 People with learning disabilities currently have little control over their own lives, though almost all, including the most severely disabled, are capable of making choices and expressing their views and preferences. The current problems are:

- Services have been too slow to recognise that people with learning disabilities have rights like other citizens;

- Provision of advocacy services is patchy;

- People with learning disabilities have little involvement in decision making;

- Few people with learning disabilities receive direct payments;

- People with learning disabilities and their families are not central to the planning process;

- Not enough effort to communicate with people with learning disabilities in accessible ways.

4.2 The challenge for public services is to find ways to give people with learning disabilities more control over their lives through:

- Developing and expanding advocacy services, particularly citizen advocacy and self-advocacy;

- Fully involving them in decisions affecting their lives;

- Increasing the number who receive direct payments;

- Developing a person-centred approach to planning services;

- Improving information and communication with people with learning disabilities.

What More Needs To Be Done

KEY ACTIONS – CHOICE AND CONTROL FOR PEOPLE WITH LEARNING DISABILITIES

- Disability Rights Commission to work for people with learning disabilities.

- £1.3 million per annum for the next three years to develop and expand advocacy services in partnership with the voluntary sector.

- Legislation to extend eligibility for direct payments supported by implementation programme to promote take up.

- Department of Health guidance to be issued in 2001 on a person-centred approach to planning services.

- Transfer of responsibility to local councils for people with preserved rights: Councils required to offer direct payments.

- The Learning Disability Development Fund will provide resources to support development of person-centred planning.

- National Forum for people with learning disabilities set up in 2001.

- Advice on involving people with learning disabilities in decision making to be issued.

- People with learning disabilities to benefit from expansion and integration of community equipment services.

Disability Rights Commission

4.3   The Disability Rights Commission will play an important role in helping individuals enforce their rights under the Disability Discrimination Act. A group is being set up to advise the Commission on issues relating to people with learning disabilities. It has drawn up a programme to ensure that the voices of people with disabilities are heard by:

- Involving them in developing the Commission's strategic plan and consultations on major policy issues;

- Producing materials in accessible formats;

- Advising the public sector and business on best practice in involving and communicating with people with learning disabilities.

4.4   The Department of Health will also work with the Commission to consider the way forward for advocacy for all disabled people.

Advocacy

4.5   Effective advocacy can transform the lives of people with learning disabilities by enabling them to express their wishes and aspirations and make real choices. Advocacy helps people put forward their views and play an active part in planning and designing services which are responsive to their needs. This applies to people with severe and profound disabilities and to the less severely disabled.

4.6   With the right support, many people with learning disabilities can become effective self-advocates. The growth of the self-advocacy movement[9] shows how people with learning disabilities can make a real difference to service development and delivery. Citizen advocates[10] make a vital contribution to enabling the voices of people with more complex disabilities to be heard.

4.7   Both citizen advocacy and self-advocacy are unevenly developed across the country. Barriers to future development include: insecure funding; limited support for local groups; and potential for conflicts of interest with statutory agencies who provide funding. This must change.

Swindon People First

Established in 1988 since 1995 this self-advocacy group has had about 120 members involved in activities such as consultation with members about the services they use; sitting on advisory panels and being members of a large Joint Working Group; interviewing managers with social services for their jobs; lay assessing and consultation with members who don't use words to communicate. They currently run a Direct Payments Support Scheme as well as a research project into how direct payments are working for people with learning disabilities across the UK. They have been very successful in obtaining funding from trusts and charities for project development and are in a promising position to build for the future.

9   Self-advocacy is people speaking up for themselves
10   Citizen advocates (ie volunteers) create a relationship with a person with learning disabilities', seeking to understand and represent the person with learning disabilities' views

4.8 The NHS Plan states that by 2002 an NHS-wide Patient and Advocacy Liaison Service (PALS) will be established in every NHS Trust, beginning with every major hospital. This will include all those Trusts offering specialist learning disability services and other health services to people with learning disabilities. PALS will be an accessible and visible service whose role will be to resolve patients', families', and carers' problems and concerns as quickly as possible. PALS will not replace external advocacy services for learning disabled people, but, where necessary, it will be able to provide signposting to independent advocacy services.

4.9 The Government's long-term aim is to have a range of independent advocacy services available in each area so that people with learning disabilities can choose the one which best meets their needs. To achieve this, we will work in partnership with citizen advocacy and self-advocacy groups to promote and sustain development of independent local advocacy schemes. We are investing at least £1.3 million for each of the next three years for this purpose. We will monitor and evaluate the impact of this funding. The new funding will be used to:

- establish a National Citizen Advocacy Network for Learning Disability led by a consortium of leading voluntary organisations. It will be charged with distributing funds to local groups in an equitable and open manner, operating within criteria drawn up after consultation with relevant interests and agreed by the Department of Health. The aim will be to work towards at least one citizen advocacy group in each local authority area. We will take steps to ensure this funding is not used to replace existing funding sources for citizen advocacy;

- increase funding for local self-advocacy groups and strengthen the national infrastructure for self-advocacy. The Department of Health will invite bids from self-advocacy groups in each of its eight regions. The Government will work in partnership with the self-advocacy movement to promote the development of a clear national voice for people with learning disabilities.

4.10 Development of, and support for, advocacy services will also be a priority area for the Learning Disability Development Fund.

4.11 People with learning disabilities from minority ethnic communities can find it particularly difficult to gain access to the advocacy support they need. The Government will ensure that our new initiatives are responsive to their needs. The Department of Health will issue good practice materials to help with this.

'The Government has got to understand how we feel about these things.' (Malcolm)

'The [advocate] explains to me what I don't understand, what social services are talking about. If I didn't understand what the questions were, she'd repeat it and explain it. She was brilliant. Helped me with debts. Had problems with money-still have problems. Calming me down when I get stressed. Any problems I tell her and she tried to help me. If I'm in bad distress I tell [her] and she tells me who to get in touch with. I've never had anyone better.' (Ruby)

Hampshire Social Services operates a flexible system to make direct payments available to people with learning disabilities. This minimises potential blocks. People have the option to purchase care from agencies rather than employing personal assistants. Existing networks support the person receiving the direct payment or, where these do not exist, arrangements are made to provide the individual support required.

Two examples

One young man, living with his parents, receives a direct payment to employ a support worker from an agency for short breaks. Breaks can be a few hours in the evening and weekends or longer. He chooses how to spend his time with the support worker and his mother has a break.

One man living with his mother wanted to move on from the day service and have more control over what he did and when. He now purchases the services of a support worker from a local agency to help him go to local leisure facilities in the evening. The local self-advocacy group, which has set up a support system for people receiving direct payments provides the support.

Direct Payments

4.12 Direct payments give local councils power to offer people money to pay for the support they have been assessed as needing in lieu of providing the services direct. The Carers and Disabled Children Act 2000 extends direct payments to carers and to disabled 16- and 17-year-olds. The Health and Social Care Bill includes provisions to extend the scope of direct payments. Subject to Parliamentary approval the legislation will:

- require local councils to make direct payments where an individual who requests and consents to one meets the criteria;

- enable local councils to make direct payments to disabled parents to meet their child's needs and for local council provided rehabilitation services.

4.13 Direct payments are highly effective in enabling people with learning disabilities to gain greater control over their lives, because they can choose how they want their support needs met. In autumn 2000 only 216 people with learning disabilities were receiving such payments out of a total of over 3,700 people. This needs to change. The provisions in the Health and Social Care Bill are intended to result in more people with learning disabilities receiving direct payments.

4.14 The success of direct payments for people with learning disabilities depends on good support services. Most local councils operate support schemes, but often these are focused on the types of support people with physical disabilities may need. Schemes must be accessible to people with learning disabilities, so that they too have the right support to manage a direct payment and remain in control. Our proposals for developing and expanding advocacy services will enable more people to access direct payments. Subject to the Health and Social Care Bill completing its passage through Parliament, the Department of Health will issue guidance on the new provisions and how people with learning disabilities can be helped to use direct payments. This will include provision of support services.

4.15 Promoting direct payments is a key element of our new vision for people with learning disabilities. The national Implementation Support Team will focus on working with local councils to achieve higher take-up. The Department of Health will consult on a performance indicator in the Personal Social Services Performance Assessment Framework.

People with Preserved Rights

4.16 People in residential care on 31 March 1993 have preserved rights to receive a higher rate of income support from which they can purchase their care. Around 30,000 are younger disabled people. Following the announcement in the NHS Plan, the Health and Social Care Bill contains provisions to transfer responsibility for their assessment and care management to local authorities. This will give this group more choice about where they live and close the shortfall in funding. The Department of Social Security will transfer resources to local authorities for their new responsibilities. Subject to Parliamentary approval these changes will come into effect in April 2002. Guidance on this change will say that councils will be required to offer the option of direct payments to anyone who meets the prescribed conditions.

A Person-Centred Approach to Planning

4.17 A person-centred approach to planning means that planning should start with the individual (not with services), and take account of their wishes and aspirations. Person-centred planning is a mechanism for reflecting the needs and preferences of a person with a learning disability and covers such issues as housing, education, employment and leisure.

4.18 Care management is the main way individuals link with services. The type and extent of care management can vary markedly between council areas. This can result in duplicated assessments and care plans for some people with learning disabilities, while others receive insufficient attention. Some people receiving publicly funded services have problems accessing the care management they need. This confusing and inconsistent situation is unacceptable.

PRIORITIES FOR PERSON-CENTRED PLANNING

4.19 The Government will issue further guidance later this year to help local councils develop a person-centred approach and put people with learning disabilities and their families at the centre of the process of planning services for and with them. We expect Learning Disability Partnership Boards to use this guidance to agree a local framework by April 2002. It will take time to develop a person-centred approach to planning for everyone who needs services. Local areas may wish to develop their own priorities, paying particular

Alan is in his 50s and now lives in his own terraced house. He wasn't happy living in a hostel nor in his own flat with support from a key worker. He met someone who was getting a direct payment and decided '– *yes that's for me! I like the idea of employing my own personal assistants who I could ask to do what I wanted when I wanted.*' His social worker put him in touch with the local independent direct payments support agency. They helped him apply for a direct payment, advertise for personal assistants and prepare job descriptions and contracts. They arranged training about direct payments and employment. Alan said '*Without the training I wouldn't have been able to cope with a direct payment.*' Now he gives talks to social workers and people with learning disabilities about how to get a direct payment.

Susan, who is in her early 20s, is severely disabled. She makes her views known through her actions, verbal responses, facial expressions and moods. Susan's circle of support realised she was unhappy with her existing services and put together a package of money to enable her to live independently. Direct payments are part of the package. The circle formed itself into a user-controlled trust fund, which manages the direct payment. Susan's expressions and views guide how the money is spent, so she is in control of the use of the money. Direct payments mean Susan can live in her own house with her own rota of support workers. She is relaxed, confident and content with a full social life and is very much part of the community.

attention to those individuals who are poorly served. However the Government also has some specific priorities. These include:

By 2003:

- People still living in long-stay hospitals;
- Young people moving from children's to adult services.

By 2004 we expect to see significant progress in the following areas:

- People using large day centres;
- People living in the family home with carers aged over 70;
- People living on NHS residential campuses.

CARE MANAGEMENT

4.20 Care management will continue to be the formal mechanism for linking individuals with public services. Its systems must be responsive to person-centred planning, and have the capacity to deliver the kinds of individualised services likely to emerge from the process. It must link effectively with other plans including:

- vocational plans (led by Connexions for young people);
- health action plans (led by an identified health professional);
- housing plans, (including a joint housing/community care assessment);
- communications plans, (where the person has communications difficulties).

4.21 Development of a person-centred approach requires real changes in organisational culture and practice. Achieving these changes should be a priority for Partnership Boards.

4.22 Given the importance of person-centred planning as a tool for achieving change, we will make supporting its implementation one of the priorities for the Learning Disability Development Fund and the Implementation Support Team. Its development and the responses of the services will be monitored, along with the extent to which person-centred services emerge as a consequence.

FAIR ACCESS TO CARE

4.23 Later in 2001 the Government will be issuing the Fair Access to Care (FACS) guidance. This will set out how eligibility for adult social care services should be determined, and following implementation from April 2002, should lead to a more consistent and fairer access to care services. The guidance will also cover procedures for reviewing adult service users' needs and continuing eligibility for support. At the same time, the Government will publish general principles of assessment to update previous 1990/1991 guidance.

4.24 In implementing this guidance councils will need to take a corporate approach, with eligibility criteria agreed across all council departments and with health and other local agencies. Councils and local health bodies will be specifically asked to develop joint eligibility criteria for adult social care and continuing health care. Partnership Boards will need to ensure that all systems are compatible with this guidance.

4.25 Person-centred frameworks will need to be fully compatible with the locally agreed joint eligibility criteria which councils and local health bodies will be asked to develop following the Fair Access to Care guidance.

INDIVIDUAL CO-ORDINATION

4.26 By July 2002 all people with learning disabilities who make substantial and long-term use of publicly funded services should have a named individual to act as their service co-ordinator. The co-ordinator will be responsible for ensuring effective organisation and monitoring of services by all relevant agencies and will be the first point of contact for people with learning disabilities and their families.

Involvement In Policy Development and Decision Making

4.27 People with learning disabilities should be fully involved in the decision making processes that affect their lives. This applies to decisions on day to day matters such as choice of activities, operational matters such as staff selection and strategic matters such as changes to eligibility criteria. It is no longer acceptable for organisations to view people with learning disabilities as passive recipients of services; they must instead be seen as active partners. Further advice will be issued in 2001 to help local agencies involve people with learning disabilities in decision making.

4.28 At national level, we have begun to involve people with learning disabilities in policy development. The Service Users Advisory Group played an important role in developing the new strategy. During 2001 the Group will develop into a more nationally

"People First has learnt a lot by being part of this Strategy Group and we hope that we can work together more in the future. **I am proud of being included in this group**.

It means a lot to me to work together with such a good team of people who are all committed to supporting people with learning difficulties in their hard struggle to live independent lives. (Carol)

representative forum linking with local groups of learning disabled people. The National Forum for People with Learning Disabilities will contribute to monitoring the impact of *Valuing People*.

4.29 *Making Decisions* (published October 1999) set out the Government's proposals to reform the law in order to improve and clarify the decision making process for those people unable to make decisions for themselves. The proposals include: definition of capacity; factors to be taken into account in assessing a person's best interest and the introduction of general authority to act reasonably which will regulate day-to-day decisions. *Making Decisions* also sets out proposals to introduce Continuing Powers of Attorney to replace Enduring Powers of Attorney, and a modernised court which will deal with all areas of decision making for adults without capacity.

Communication and Equipment

4.30 The Government expects organisations working with learning disabled people to develop communication policies and produce and disseminate information in accessible formats. For those with severe disabilities this may require individual communication techniques and effective use of new technology.

4.31 People with learning disabilities may need specialist equipment because they also have a physical disability or sensory impairment. Assistive technology can increase their control, choice and independence through improving cognitive and social functioning. It can also enable people with learning disabilities to make good use of education, training and employment opportunities. From April 2001 councils with social services responsibilities and the NHS will receive additional funding to improve and expand community equipment services. By 2004 the Government expects health and social services to integrate their community equipment services, and increase by 50% the number of people benefiting from them.

CHAPTER 5

SUPPORTING CARERS

Government Objective: To increase the help and support carers receive from all local agencies in order to fulfil their family and caring roles effectively.

This Chapter focuses on the rights of carers. Carers need to be confident that public services will provide reliable support for their family members with learning disabilities, and that our proposals for improving services will bring them benefits. The support and commitment of carers is critical in enabling people with learning disabilities to achieve independence, choice and inclusion.

Problems and Challenges

5.1 Caring for a family member with a learning disability is a lifelong commitment, which continues even when the person is living away from the family home. Carers make a vital contribution to the lives of people with learning disabilities, often providing most of the support they need. They are a crucial resource for ensuring that people with learning disabilities can live in the community. We have no precise data on numbers, but it is estimated that some 60% of adults with learning disabilities live with their families. Statutory agencies do not always properly recognise the extent of carers' contribution or its value.

5.2 Carers face many problems and challenges. They need:

● More and better information;

● Better assessment of their own needs;

● Improved access to support services such as day services and short break services (respite care) particularly for those with more severe disabilities;

● To be treated as valued partners by local agencies, not as barriers to their son's or daughter's greater independence.

5.3 The challenge is to ensure that carers:

- receive the right support to help them in their caring role;

- obtain relevant information about services;

- know who to approach for advice and help;

- are respected and treated as individuals in their own right;

- make their voices heard at national and local level.

What More Needs To Be Done

KEY ACTIONS – CARERS

- Carers of people with learning disabilities to benefit from all mainstream carers initiatives.

- Implementation of Carers and Disabled Children Act 2000.

- In partnership with Mencap the Government will provide £250,000 per annum for the next three years to develop a National Learning Disability Information Centre and Help Line.

- New guidance on exclusions from services.

- Local councils to pay particular attention to identifying and supporting carers aged over 70 and carers from minority ethnic communities.

- Carers and carer organisations to be represented on Learning Disability Task Force.

National Carers Strategy

5.4 The Government is determined to improve support for carers. *Caring about Carers: the Report of the National Carers Strategy* sets out our general approach. Social security benefits are being increased to help carers. From April 2001 a package of extra support worth £500 million over the next three years will help some 300,000 carers. We are increasing the carer premium in income related benefits by 70% (from £14.15 to £24.40). We are also raising the earnings limit (now £50 per week) in the Invalid Care Allowance (ICA) to the level of Lower Earnings Limit (currently £67 per week). Subject to a suitable legislative opportunity we will extend the opportunity to claim ICA to people aged 65 and over and the entitlement to ICA for up to 8 weeks after the death of the disabled person will also help carers.

5.5 The Government expects carers of people with learning disabilities to benefit from all mainstream carer initiatives. This requires effective targeting at local and national levels. Carers must be able to obtain information, advice and help easily from local agencies, especially local councils with social services responsibilities and must be given a single point of contact.

Implementation of the Carers and Disabled Children Act 2000

5.6 The Carers and Disabled Children Act 2000 comes into force in April 2001. It extends a carer's right to an assessment, already provided for in the Carers and Recognition and Services Act 1995, to carers where the person cared for has refused an assessment or has refused community care services, and gives local councils the power to offer carers services to support them in their caring role and to help them maintain their own health and well being. The Department of Health is issuing guidance to local councils on implementing the legislation together with a leaflet *The Carers Guide to a Carer's Assessment* to be made available to all carers. The Government is committed to ensuring that these new rights become a reality. We shall consult on a new Performance Indicator to monitor how many people with learning disabilities are receiving breaks services (respite care).

Excluding People from Services

5.7 Excluding people with learning disabilities from services if they are found to be difficult to handle or present with challenging behaviour represents a major cause of stress for carers, who may be left unsupported to cope with their son or daughter at home. This practice is unacceptable and families must not be left to cope unaided. No service should be withdrawn on these grounds without identifying alternative options and putting a suitable alternative service in place where possible. Decisions to exclude a person with learning disabilities from a service should always be referred to the Learning Disability Partnership Board, which will be responsible for the provision of alternative services in such cases, provided the person meets the eligibility criteria. This issue will be addressed in the guidance to be issued on implementing *Valuing People*.

Tameside: Flexible Respite Services

Three years ago the council identified money within the learning disability budget to develop an alternative option to the building based respite service. A flexible service has now been developed to support people in their own homes or in accessing community services and provide a break for carers. People access it for between 1 or 2 hours and 10 hours a week, which has opened up many opportunities for people to go to community facilities with individual support. Last year the council used money from the Carers Grant and the Promoting Independence Grant to expand the service. It now provides 340–350 hours a month to around 36 people. The independent sector provides the service: about 90% is delivered by the same provider who runs the building based respite care service.

Information for Carers

5.8   Carers need more and better information provided in ways that are easily accessible. The most effective information exchange is often between carers, who share experiences and solutions. These networks also need reliable information from others. Many organisations provide telephone and written advice, but there is currently no national Information Centre or Help Line for people needing help on learning disability issues.

5.9   In order to fill this gap, the Department of Health is providing £750,000 over the next 3 years to enable Mencap to work with other key interests to establish a National Learning Disability Information Centre and telephone help and advice line. The Centre will provide help to all who need it, including people with learning disabilities and professionals, but we expect it to have a particularly important role for carers. Services to be provided will include:

*   Advice on all aspects of learning disability and the services and help people with learning disabilities need;

*   Links and collaboration with the Contact a Family Information Centre for Children (see paragraph 3.12);

*   Links with other databases and websites, including the National Electronic Library for Health, the Social Care Institute of Excellence, and NHS Direct on line;

*   Putting people in touch with local support groups.

The Carers Grant: Meeting the Needs of Older Carers and Carers from Minority Ethnic Communities

5.10   *Family Matters, Counting Families In* published alongside *Valuing People* identifies three groups of carers who face additional pressures: older carers (those aged 70 or over), carers from minority ethnic communities and carers whose sons or daughters are going through transition from school to adult life. Chapter 3 looks at transition, and we discuss below the other two priority groups. Both face additional difficulties in carrying out their caring role effectively.

5.11   It is estimated that a third of people with learning disabilities living in the family home are living with a carer aged 70 or over. Many are sole carers with reduced support. In many cases the learning disabled person also takes on a caring role, but this is not generally recognised and they are often not properly supported. There is some evidence to suggest that up to 25% of people with learning disabilities do not become known to statutory agencies until later in life, when the parent becomes too frail to continue caring for their adult son or daughter. Lack of planning for the future creates anxiety and stress for the parent and the learning disabled person. This group is one of the priority groups for developing a person-centred approach to planning (see paragraph 4.19). We propose to introduce a Performance Indicator: % of carers aged 70 or over for whom a plan has been agreed. This will be monitored as part of the arrangements for monitoring the White Paper.

5.12 Difficulties facing carers from minority ethnic communities include insensitivity to issues of culture and language and false assumptions about communities wishing to provide care within their own family environment or putting up barriers against statutory agencies. All services for carers should be responsive to the needs of people from minority ethnic communities.

5.13 The Carers Grant provides funds to help ensure that substantial and regular carers, who will include lifelong carers, get a break from caring when they need it. Analysis of the Grant's first year of operation (1999/2000) shows that at least 10% of the total grant of £20 million was spent on breaks for carers of adults with learning disabilities. Over the next 3 years the amount available for all carers will be £70 million/£85 million/£100 million.

5.14 The Department of Health will shortly issue new guidance for the Carers Grant 2001/02 which will encourage local councils to identify older carers and carers from minority ethnic communities.

5.15 The Department of Health will monitor the impact of its new guidelines as part of the process of monitoring the Grant. People living with carers aged 70 or over will also be an early priority for the introduction of person-centred planning.

Carers as Partners

5.16 It is essential that the voices of carers are clearly heard in policy development and implementation at both national and local levels. Carers should be treated as full partners by all agencies involved. The Government will ensure that carers are represented on the Learning Disability Task Force. We will also ensure that this group of carers contributes to the Department of Health's existing arrangements for discussing policy and practice issues with the generic national carers' organisations. We expect this to be mirrored at local level so that carers participate in debates about local policy development.

5.17 Carers have training needs and can also be a training resource. Local councils should offer them training opportunities so that they develop their skills. Professional staff can learn a great deal from their experience and expertise. The Government will require local agencies to ensure that carers and their organisations are fully involved in the development of local action plans for implementing the White Paper.

CHAPTER 6

IMPROVING HEALTH FOR PEOPLE WITH LEARNING DISABILITIES

Government Objective: To enable people with learning disabilities to access a health service designed around their individual needs, with fast and convenient care delivered to a consistently high standard, and with additional support where necessary.

This chapter shows how the Government's commitment in the NHS Plan to a person-centred health service which challenges discrimination on all grounds will improve health care for people with learning disabilities. Good health is an essential prerequisite for achieving independence, choice and inclusion.

Problems and challenges

6.1 Most people with learning disabilities have greater health needs than the rest of the population. They are more likely to experience mental illness and are more prone to chronic health problems, epilepsy, and physical and sensory disabilities. An increasing number of young people with severe and profound disabilities have complex health needs. Poor oral health may lead to chronic dental disease. As life expectancy increases age-related diseases such as stroke, heart disease, chronic respiratory disease and cancer are likely to be of particular concern. There is an above average death rate among younger people with learning disabilities.

6.2 Surveys have highlighted shortfalls in primary care and hospital provision. *Facing the Facts*, for example, found inconsistencies in the provision of health care in different parts of the country. When people with learning disabilities approached health care providers for assessment or treatment they often found difficulties in gaining access to the help they needed. The health needs of people with learning disabilities may not be recognised by doctors and care staff who have no experience of working with people who have difficulties in communication. Health outcomes for people with learning disabilities fall short when compared with outcomes for the non-disabled population. We know that:

- Few people with learning disabilities access health screening services with uptake rates for breast and cervical screening being especially poor.

- Research has highlighted inadequate diagnosis and treatment of specific medical conditions, including heart disease, hypothyroidism and osteoporosis.

- Studies of the management of people with challenging behaviour has shown an over-dependence on the use of psychotropic drugs with poor outcomes as a consequence.

- Doctors and care staff can fail to recognise the potential health complications of many of the conditions that cause learning disability.

6.3 Because mainstream health services have been slow in developing the capacity and skills to meet the needs of people with learning disabilities, some NHS specialist learning disability services have sought to provide all encompassing services on their own. As a result the wider NHS has failed to consider the needs of people with learning disabilities. This is the most important issue which the NHS needs to address for people with learning disabilities.

What More Needs To Be Done

KEY ACTIONS – HEALTH

- Action to reduce health inequalities: explore feasibility of establishing a confidential inquiry into mortality among people with learning disabilities.

- Action to challenge discrimination against people with learning disabilities from minority ethnic communities.

- Health facilitators identified for people with learning disabilities by Spring 2003.

- All people with a learning disability to be registered with a GP by June 2004.

- All people with a learning disability to have a Health Action Plan by June 2005.

- NHS to ensure that all mainstream hospital services are accessible to people with learning disabilities.

- Development of local specialist services for people with severe challenging behaviour to be a priority for the capital element of the Learning Disability Development Fund.

- Mental Health NSF will bring new benefits to people with learning disabilities.

- New role for specialist learning disability services, making most effective use of their expertise.

Reducing Health Inequalities

6.4   The NHS Plan made clear that inequalities in health cannot be tackled without dealing with the fundamental causes – including poverty, low educational attainment, unemployment, discrimination and social exclusion. These factors affect many people with learning disabilities, and their high morbidity and mortality rates show the importance of addressing their needs. The Government has launched a comprehensive plan to tackle health inequalities and work is taking place across Government to tackle the root causes.

6.5   The Government has announced that local health inequalities targets will be reinforced by the creation of national health inequalities targets, to be delivered by a combination of specific health policies and broader Government policies. Health policies such as improved access to services, smoking cessation, healthy diet and exercise will be particularly important for narrowing the gap between the health of learning disabled people and the population as a whole. In addition, health authorities should take account of the needs of learning disabled people in planning services and making them accessible to all.

6.6 Those who live and work with people with learning disabilities are well placed to encourage healthier life styles. Providers of support in social care settings have a responsibility for ensuring that an individual's general health needs are met, by developing links with health professionals, promoting family and staff competence in basic health issues and implementing health promotion initiatives.

6.7 The Government will ensure that policies on health inequality make explicit reference to people with learning disabilities. Health Action Zones, for example, should ensure that the needs of people with learning disabilities are being addressed within their areas when undertaking work to meet the needs of vulnerable people. Successful innovative learning disability work being led by HAZs should be identified and highlighted so that this can be mainstreamed and replicated elsewhere. Health Improvement Plans (HimPs) will provide a means of addressing the health needs of people with learning disabilities so that they do not experience avoidable illness and premature death.

6.8 Evidence of avoidable illness and premature death amongst people with learning disabilities is a major cause of concern for the Government. We will explore the feasibility of establishing a confidential inquiry into mortality among people with learning disabilities. This will help us take steps to reduce the number of avoidable deaths.

6.9 The Government will explore the possibility of developing performance indicators to compare the health status of the learning disabilities population with that of the general population. We shall consult on performance indicators later this year.

People with learning disabilities from minority ethnic communities

6.10 People with learning disabilities from minority ethnic communities are at particular risk of discrimination in gaining access to appropriate health care. Problems arise if professionals are not aware of cultural or language issues or only use English language based assessment tools. The NHS Plan recognises that ethnic minorities can face discrimination in gaining access to health services and confirms the Government's commitment to tackling the problem. Achieving this will be helped by the new statutory duty to promote race equality, in the Race Relations (Amendment) Act 2000. From 2 April 2001 listed public bodies, including central and local Government, the NHS and NHS Trusts, for example, will be obliged to work towards the elimination of unlawful racial discrimination and to promote good relations between persons of different racial groups. Staff who understand the values and concerns of minority ethnic communities and who can communicate effectively with them have an important role to play in ensuring that minority ethnic communities can access the health care they need.

Meeting Health Needs

6.11 For most people, GPs, practice nurses and other members of primary care teams provide the main contact with the NHS. In future, we expect this to be the same for people with learning disabilities. Building on the guidance on good practice in primary care given in *Once A Day*, the primary care team will play a key role in providing health care for people with learning disabilities and in ensuring that people with learning disabilities can access the full range of health services to meet both their ordinary health needs and their additional health requirements through referral to specialist services. Primary care teams also have a key role in supporting and improving the health of carers.

Health Facilitators

6.12 As the first point of contact, primary care is the place where many important decisions are made. But for many people with learning disabilities their encounter with the primary care team may be frustrating and difficult. In order to overcome these barriers staff from the local community learning disability team in each area will need to take on the role of health facilitators to support people with learning disabilities to access the health care they need from primary care and other NHS services. This role might be taken up by any community learning disability team member, but learning disability nurses will be well placed to fulfil this role.

Primary health care in Liverpool

'Speaking up' in public to doctors and nurses at a Primary Care Group Board was a new experience for self-advocates from the Toxteth and Granby Resource Centre, Liverpool. Some of the things they said were:

'We would like the same checks as everyone else'

'We want – you to explain and listen to us and not just talk to our carers; leaflets about health with pictures and get to know us as people and ask our point of view.'

The result was an agreement to review primary care provision across the area.'

6.13 Health facilitators will help general practitioners and others in the primary care team to identify their patients with learning disabilities, in collaboration with colleagues from social services, education and health. Their task will be to facilitate, to advocate and to ensure that people with learning disabilities gain full access to the health care they need, whether from primary or secondary NHS services. The role of the health facilitators should embrace mental as well as physical needs. The health facilitator role will be vital in helping people with learning disabilities navigate their way around the health service.

6.14 All people with learning disabilities should be registered with a general practitioner. We expect that all general practices, with support from the health facilitator and in partnership with specialist learning disability services, will have identified all people with a learning disability registered with the practice by June 2004. Progress in achieving this objective will be monitored by the Department of Health.

Health Action Plans

Anna has Down's syndrome. She uses a wheelchair and cannot communicate verbally. Her support team had difficulty in involving her in planning as she was lethargic, passive and difficult to motivate. A health care check revealed that she had undiagnosed thyroid problems, diabetes and hypertension. After treatment Anna became more involved, used her wheelchair less, and volunteered to help in a children's day centre.

6.15 The Government expects each individual with a learning disability to be offered a personal Health Action Plan (HAP). Responsibility for ensuring completion of the HAP will rest with the health facilitator in partnership with primary care nurses and general practitioners. The HAP will form part of the person-centred plan. The HAP is an action plan and will include details of the need for health interventions, oral health and dental care, fitness and mobility, continence, vision, hearing, nutrition and emotional needs as well as details of medication taken, side effects, and records of any screening tests.

6.16 Health Action Plans will be offered and reviewed at the following stages of peoples' lives:

- Transition from secondary education with a process for ongoing referral;
- Leaving home to move into a residential service;
- Moving home from one provider to another;
- Moving to an out of area placement;
- Changes in health status, for example as a result of a period of out-patient care or in-patient treatment;
- On retirement;
- When planning transition for those living with older family carers.

6.17 The Government expects all Learning Disability Partnership Boards to have agreed a framework for the introduction of Health Action Plans and to have ensured that there are clearly identified health facilitators for all people with learning disability by June 2003. All people with learning disabilities should have a HAP by June 2005.

6.18 Primary Care Trusts in their commissioning role should ensure that general health care for people with learning disabilities is built into existing priorities. Partnership Boards need to work with the Primary Care Trusts to ensure that there is an integrated plan for supporting the primary and general health care services to work with people with learning disabilities, with clarity about expectations upon both general practice and general hospitals.

Secondary health care

6.19 Mainstream secondary health services must also be accessible for people with learning disabilities. There must be no discrimination. Support will be needed to help people with learning disabilities admitted to a general hospital for medical or surgical treatment to help them to understand and co-operate in their treatment. The NHS will ensure that all its procedures comply with the Disability Discrimination Act and that its staff recruitment and training practices are also fully compliant. Whenever possible NHS resources should be used to provide the appropriate health care support to enable people to live in their own home.

6.20 Health facilitators will have primary responsibility for facilitating access to secondary health care. But by 2002 a Patient Advocacy and Liaison Service (PALS) will be established in every NHS Trust. Individuals will then have an identifiable person they can turn to if they have a problem or need information while they are using hospital and other NHS services. Within the 130 or more NHS Trusts providing specialist health care for people with learning disabilities, PALS will have an especially important role for ensuring that people with learning disabilities can access the full range of NHS provision. PALS will complement the work of the health facilitator.

Consent to Treatment

6.21 The Government is committed to having good consent to treatment practice in place in all health settings. This is of particular importance in general hospitals where staff may be unfamiliar with seeking consent from people who have learning disabilities. The

Specialist Learning Disability Services

6.27 It is essential that sufficient good quality multi-disciplinary specialist services are available to meet the needs of people with learning disabilities. Locally based specialist community learning disability services are key components of the modern NHS. Over 130 NHS Trusts in England provide specialist services for people with learning disabilities. Through these NHS Trusts people with learning disabilities have access to a range of learning disability specialists including learning disability nurses, occupational therapists, physiotherapists, psychiatrists, speech and language therapists and clinical psychologists, working in a multi-disciplinary way in close collaboration with social workers and care managers. Other NHS professionals such as dieticians, psychotherapists and creative therapists, chiropodists, opticians, audiologists and pharmacists also have specialist roles.

6.28 The Government believes that professional staff employed in locally based specialist services provide vital support for people with learning disabilities. But their role must change. Staff may continue to work within specialist clinical directorates, but their tasks will need to be refocused to give greater emphasis to their role in providing high quality specialist expertise. They will also take on a key supplementary role in supporting people to access mainstream services.

6.29 Specialist services should be planned and delivered with a focus on the whole person, ensuring continuity of provision and appropriate partnership between different agencies and professions. To support these aims, services will need to demonstrate that they are listening carefully to the views and experiences of people with learning disabilities and their families, which should also play a critical part in the education and training of paid staff.

6.30 In their specialist role staff should recognise the importance of enhancing the competence of local services to enable service users to remain in their usual surroundings and save the often high costs (both personal and financial) of specialist placements out of area. Specialist staff will need to give more time to facilitating the work of others in mainstream services to developing the capacity of services to support those with complex needs to service design and less to direct interventions. Partnership Boards will review the role of specialist learning disability services to bring them into line with the new vision outlined here.

6.31 In addition to their clinical and therapeutic roles specialist staff should take on the following complementary tasks:

- a health promotion role; working closely with the local health promotion team;

- a health facilitation role; working with primary care teams, community health professionals and staff involved in delivering secondary health care;

- a teaching role; to enable a wide range of staff, including those who work in social services and the independent sector, to become more familiar with how to support people with learning disabilities to have their health needs met;

- A service development role; contributing their knowledge of health issues to planning processes.

Intensive Health Care Support

6.32 A proportion of people with learning disabilities will require intensive health care support through specialist community services, including learning disability teams and/or challenging behaviour teams, over a prolonged period of time – because of their complex disability or the challenges they place on services. Such people have the same entitlements to independence, choice, inclusion and civil rights as all others. The aim should be to provide them with ordinary housing and support services, in the least restrictive environment possible, with opportunities to lead full and purposeful lives.

6.33 Many people with such complex needs are currently living in community services as NHS in-patients. This is only appropriate where people require continuous medical supervision. A need for nursing supervision is not a sufficient reason for NHS in-patient care. Localities with large numbers of people living in such NHS accommodation should use person-centred planning and pooled budgets to design more appropriate locally based housing and support and so reduce the number of long term NHS in-patient beds to more appropriate levels. Forthcoming guidance on continuing care from the Department of Health will support this approach.

CHAPTER 7

HOUSING, FULFILLING LIVES AND EMPLOYMENT

This chapter sets out the Government's programme for reform in three areas which are of central importance in the lives of all people with learning disabilities: housing, living a fulfilling life, and employment. Bringing about change in all these areas will be essential in order to achieve greater independence, choice and inclusion for people with learning disabilities.

HOUSING

Government objective: To enable people with learning disabilities and their families to have greater choice and control over where and how they live.

Problems and Challenges

David inherited the tenancy of a housing association bungalow following his mother's death. He has a support package from a care provider and had some intensive support from the Community Team for Learning Disabilities to improve his cooking and domestic skills. His brother and sister-in-law live nearby and provide emotional and practical support. He is now coping well.

7.1 Most people with learning disabilities live with their families. Often they leave the family home only as the result of a crisis such as the illness or death of the carer. Planning ahead to move to more independent living is not always possible as the appropriate housing, care and support options may not be available. With growing numbers of people living with older carers, the Government wishes to see better forward planning by local councils so that carers do not face continuing uncertainty in old age and their sons and daughters gain greater independence in a planned way.

7.2 People with learning disabilities can live successfully in different types of housing, from individual self-contained properties, housing networks, group homes, and shared accommodation schemes, through to village and other forms of intentional community. They can cope with the full range of tenures, including home ownership.

Expanding the range and choice of housing, care and support services is key to giving individuals more choice and control over their lives.

7.3   Few areas offer a full range of options. Obstacles include:

●   A culture of professionals deciding what is good for individuals, and the traditional "take what you are given" attitude in public provision of housing;

●   A conservatism in developing housing options for people with learning disabilities, with authorities replicating current provision rather than taking opportunities to broaden the range of housing available.

7.4   We now know more about outcomes associated with living in different types of accommodation. Research commissioned by the Department of Health examined the differences in cost and benefits between dispersed housing, NHS residential campuses, and village communities.[11] It found dispersed housing and village communities had strengths and weaknesses: dispersed housing was associated with greater personal choice, greater participation in community activities, wider personal relationships, and better qualified and more senior staff; village communities were associated with better activity planning, more routine day activities, better access to health checks, and less likelihood of exposure to crime or verbal abuse. There were many areas where no significant difference was found, including cost. Living in NHS residential campuses produced significantly poorer outcomes.

7.5   Various studies showed that housing design on its own does not guarantee positive outcomes. Factors such as management style and staff training are at least as important. In view of this, the Government wishes to encourage development of a range of housing options and, thus, provide real choice to people with learning disabilities and their families. No housing solution should be routinely disregarded as a matter of deliberate policy. The role of public services is to facilitate choice, not frustrate it.

7.6   Widening the housing, care and support options available creates the potential for choice, but individuals also need accessible information in order to make choices. Many people with learning disabilities will need advice and support to do this.

11 The Quality and Costs of Residential Support for People with Learning Disabilities, Summary & Implications (Hester Adrian Research Centre, University of Manchester, 1999

What More Needs To Be Done

KEY ACTIONS – HOUSING

- Housing and social services to work together to expand housing, care and support options: Department of Health and Department of the Environment, Transport and the Regions to issue new joint guidance in 2001.

- Legislation to introduce new duty on local housing authorities to provide advice and information.

- Learning Disability Partnership Boards to develop local housing strategies for people with learning disabilities.

- Learning Disability Development Fund will prioritise "supported living" approaches for people living with older carers.

- Enabling people living in the remaining long-stay hospitals to move to more appropriate accommodation by 2004 will be a priority for the Learning Disability Development Fund.

Options and Choices – Barnet

Housing and social services work together and benefit from this joint working. Social services keep an up to date list of priority cases for housing and accommodation needs. An annual quota for nominations for housing association or council lettings was jointly managed with the housing department agreeing eligibility for housing. By 1999 this had changed the range of services from one which was predominantly registered residential care to one where more than a hundred people had their own tenancy and were receiving housing benefit.

Expanding Choice in Housing, Care and Support Services

7.7 The Housing Green Paper (April 2000) set out the Government's agenda for improving the quality and choice of housing available to all. Its proposals, such as more open housing access and choice based lettings procedures, apply as much to people with learning disabilities as to other people. We are also removing other obstacles and barriers to expanding housing, care and support options by putting in place new policies and tools to create the environment and the imperative for local action.

7.8 Local housing authorities have a key role to play through their work to develop and implement local housing strategies and by providing housing advice and improving access to housing. However, they can only succeed in expanding the housing choices available to people with learning disabilities by working in partnership with social services, health and other local agencies.

7.9 In order to strengthen such partnerships, the Department of Health and the Department of the Environment, Transport and the Regions will shortly issue a joint circular and detailed guidance on commissioning the range of housing, care and support services required to expand housing choice. This will include consideration of ways to develop new joint performance indicators for social services and housing authorities.

7.10 In England there are over 4 million existing homes in the social rented sector alone. These, together with private sector housing, are potential resources that can be drawn on to open up housing, care and support options for people with learning disabilities. The Government is also making available over £10 billion of housing capital resources over the next three years to be drawn upon to finance remodelling of existing housing or new development.

7.11 The Government expects local councils to give people with learning disabilities a genuine opportunity to choose between housing, care and support options that include:

- **Supported living:** this approach is concerned with designing services round the particular needs and wishes of individuals and is less likely to result in housing and support that is designed around congregate living. Department of Health research has shown that supported living is associated with people having greater overall choice and a wider range of community activities.

- **Small scale ordinary housing:** Department of Health research has shown that small scale ordinary housing is likely to lead to better outcomes across a range of factors than is large housing or hostel provision.

- **Village and intentional communities:** These comprise houses and some shared facilities on one or more sites. Department of Health research shows such communities were associated with better activity planning, more routine day activities and better access to health checks. A study commissioned as part of the White Paper's development found 3,000 people living in 73 village and intentional communities. This study and *Facing the Facts* also indicated that some local authorities are reluctant to support people with learning disabilities who wish to live, or whose families make arrangements for them to live, in a village or intentional community.

7.12 The Government will issue statutory guidance to local councils to ensure they do not rule out any of these options when considering the future housing, care and support needs of people with learning disabilities and their families.

Supporting People

7.13 *Supporting People* is a new policy and funding framework for support services that will be implemented in April 2003. It will bring together resources from several existing programmes into a new grant to local authorities, which can be applied more flexibly to fund support services for people with learning disabilities and for other vulnerable people wherever they live. Local social services and housing authorities, working with other partners including the NHS, will be expected to establish joint arrangements for deciding how to apply the new grant and to integrate the planning and commissioning of support services with the planning and commissioning of housing, care, and health services.

Housing Advice and Assistance

7.14 Legislation to enable local authorities to introduce choice based letting systems for access to social housing is currently before Parliament. The provisions include a new duty on local housing authorities to provide assistance to people, including those with learning disabilities, who need help when applying for and obtaining social housing. Local authorities will have flexibility as to how this is provided, and how far they integrate it with their wider advice and advocacy services for people with learning disabilities.

Local Housing Strategies

7.15 Learning Disability Partnership Boards will be expected to ensure that they set out plans for the provision of information, advice and advocacy services covering the different aspects of individuals' needs, including housing, as part of the Learning Disability Joint Investment Plan (JIP). This requires the participation of housing authorities in the development of the Learning Disability JIP, and in the planning and development of services. Likewise, social services and the NHS need to be involved in developing the local housing strategy and Housing Investment Programmes. At operational level, links need to be made between local housing authorities' housing advice services and local arrangements for accessing housing, and wider person-centred planning processes for people with learning disabilities. Joint Investment Plans provide an opportunity for all stakeholders to review the housing care and support options available in their area and develop plans for how to expand choice for individuals.

People Living with Older Carers

7.16 The Government recognises that there is particular concern about the position of people with learning disabilities living with older carers aged 70 and over. They and their families need to be able to plan for the future in good time. We have therefore decided to make promoting supported living for this group of people with learning disabilities one of the priorities both the revenue and capital elements of the Learning Disability Development Fund.

The NHS as Housing Provider

7.17 For almost 30 years, successive Governments have been committed to the reprovision of long-stay hospital accommodation in order to enable people to live in community-based housing. However, there remain over 1500 people living in old long-stay hospitals. In some areas, the long-stay hospitals have been partly replaced by NHS residential campuses often on former hospital sites or in NHS homes in the community. There are about 1500 people, outside the hospitals, who remain as patients under the care of a consultant in the NHS. Research has raised significant concerns about the quality of life enjoyed by people living in NHS residential campuses developed as a result of the contraction or closure of NHS hospitals.

7.18 While people with learning disabilities, like other people, may need to be admitted to hospital on a short-term basis, we do not believe it is right for them to live in NHS hospital accommodation on a long-term basis. The Government will enable all people currently living in long-stay hospitals to move into more appropriate accommodation by April 2004. Learning Disability Partnership Boards should therefore work together to agree and implement alternative housing, care and support plans for such people in order to achieve closure of those hospitals by this date. This will be a priority for the revenue element of the Learning Disability Development Fund.

7.19 In the case of residential campuses and retained beds, Partnership Boards should agree a timetable for extending person-centred planning (to commence by October 2002) to all people currently living there. This will inform discussions with the person and their family to decide whether alternative community-based housing, care and support options would be in their best interests. Where they are, these alternatives should be made available. Where people wish to remain in NHS residential campuses, Partnership Boards will be expected to monitor and improve the quality of care they receive.

FULFILLING LIVES

Government Objective: To enable people with learning disabilities to lead full and purposeful lives within their community and to develop a range of friendships, activities and relationships.

Problems and Challenges

7.20 At present many people with learning disabilities do not take part in community activities or participate in wider social networks with non-disabled people. Few have friends apart from those paid to be with them, their close family, or other people with learning disabilities with whom they live. Being part of the local community benefits everyone. This chapter sets out the action the Government will take to help promote social inclusion for people with learning disabilities.

KEY ACTIONS – FULFILLING LIVES

- Five year programme to modernise day services by 2006 – priority for the Learning Disability Development Fund.

- Learning and Skills Council to ensure equal access to education.

- Action to outlaw discrimination against people with learning disabilities on public transport.

- Leisure plans to incorporate the needs of people with learning disabilities.

- New initiatives to improve services for parents with a learning disability

- Improved disability awareness training for Department of Social Security staff administering Disability Living Allowance.

Modernising Day Services

7.21 For decades, services for people with learning disabilities have been heavily reliant on large, often institutional, day centres. These have provided much needed respite for families, but they have made a limited contribution to promoting social inclusion or independence for people with learning disabilities. People with learning disabilities attending them have not had opportunities to develop individual interests or the skills and experience they need in order to move into employment.

7.22 Local councils currently spend over £300 million a year on day services of which more than 80% goes on over 60,000 day centre places that often focus on large, group activities. The most severely disabled people often receive the poorest service and the particular cultural needs of people from minority ethnic communities are too often not addressed.

7.23 Some local councils have done much to modernise their day services, but overall progress has been too slow. The barriers standing in the way of change include:

- Difficulties in releasing resources tied up in buildings and staff;

- Slow development of links with other services (including supported employment) and support in the wider community;

- Tension between providing respite for families and fulfilling opportunities for the person;

- Slow progress in introducing person-centred approaches to planning.

7.24 The Government wishes to see a greater emphasis on individualised and flexible services which will:

- Support people in developing their capacity to do what they want;

- Help people develop social skills and the capacity to form friendships and relationships with a wider range of people;

- Enable people to develop skills and enhance their employability;

- Help communities welcome people with learning disabilities.

7.25 These problems will be addressed through a five year programme to support local councils in modernising their day services. Our aim will be to ensure that the resources currently committed to day centres are focused on providing people with learning disabilities with new opportunities to lead full and purposeful lives. Securing the active involvement of people with learning disabilities and their families in redesigning services will be essential to the success of the programme. The Government recognises that, for many families, day centres have provided essential respite from the day to day demands of caring. The services that replace them must result in improvements for both users and their families. The needs of people with profound or complex disabilities will be carefully considered as part of the modernisation programme.

Sawston and Bottisham, Cambridgeshire

A group of people with learning disabilities won the bid to keep the vending machines in the local college filled. Another group bid to win the contract to keep the village tidy. A strong partnership with the Village College in Sawston provided a base and opportunities to participate in a range of courses. A local charity funded a job coach, so people had opportunities for individualised employment. This meant that people did not have to be bused into Cambridge to a large day centre.

7.26 Modernising day services will involve developing and strengthening links with local supported employment schemes, and with providers of further and community education and training for disabled people. The Government recognises the need to strengthen these relationships further at national level.

7.27 Day services should be modernised by 2006. Learning Disability Partnership Boards will be required to draw up modernisation programmes by 2002 for achieving this. Plans will address the future role of existing large day centres. The introduction of person-centred planning for people using day centres will be a key element for achieving this. People using them should be an early priority for person-centred planning.

7.28 Modernising day centres will be one of the priority areas for the Learning Disability Development Fund, in order to provide bridging finance to support change. The Implementation Support Team will give early priority to supporting day service modernisation.

Education and Lifelong Learning

7.29 Many people with learning disabilities make use of further education provision, Local Education Authority adult and community education and adult work-based training opportunities to develop and extend their skills. They need to have the same access as other people to opportunities for education and lifelong learning.

7.30 We recognise the importance of meeting the learning needs of people with learning disabilities through a person-centred approach. Young people in particular should not be sent to further education colleges because there is a lack of suitable provision either in updated training facilities or in supported employment. The Learning and Skills Act 2000 gives the Learning and Skills Council (LSC) specific responsibility to have regard to the needs of young people and adults with learning disabilities when securing post-16 education and training. The LSC is required to:

- Make arrangements to ensure that young people and adults with learning disabilities have access to provision which meets their needs and, where appropriate, to additional support;

- Build equality of opportunity into its policies, programmes and actions, working closely with key equality organisations including the Disability Rights Commission;

- Have regard to the needs of learners with learning difficulties when providing work experience.

The Department for Education and Employment will be working with Skill, the National Bureau for Students with Disabilities, to prepare a statement of good practice on the practical steps institutions should take to enable students to gain access to suitable places and successful work experience there.

7.31 In addition, the Government has announced that £172 million in the post-16 sector (Further Education, Higher Education, Adult Education and the Youth Service) will be used over the period 2002/03 to 2003/04 to improve accessibility for disabled students and adult learners in England. The new Adult Basic Skills Strategy Unit, based in the Department for Education and Employment, will oversee literacy and numeracy developments at national and regional level and act as a catalyst to initiate action by others to improve people's basic skills. The Unit is funding a £1.5 million project to develop ways of improving literacy and numeracy among people with learning difficulties and/or disabilities.

7.32 The Learning And Skills Act 2000 also established Local Learning Partnerships which will have a key role to promote learning and ensure it meets the needs of local communities. These Partnerships will ensure:

- effective consultative mechanisms are in place so that the views of people with learning disabilities are heard by providers and the LSC;

- the content of and access to local learning provision meet the needs of people with learning disabilities.

7.33 The Special Educational Needs and Disability Bill currently before Parliament will remove the current exemption of education from disability rights legislation and give people with disabilities new rights in Local Education Authority (LEA) adult and community education, further education, higher education institutions and LEA youth service provision. It aims to ensure that disabled students, including those with learning disabilities, are not treated less favourably than non-disabled students. Post-16 institutions will have to make reasonable adjustments to their premises to ensure that disabled students are not put at a substantial disadvantage to their peers. The Bill will make it unlawful for institutions to discriminate against disabled people not only in the way they carry out their main business – the provision of education – but also in arranging admissions and providing wider services, such as accommodation, welfare services, and careers advice.

Transport

7.34 Access to transport is essential to enable people with learning disabilities to lead full and purposeful lives. However, they currently face many obstacles using public or private transport. Transport staff and operators may not understand their needs and people may lack the necessary support and training to become independent travellers.

7.35 The Department of the Environment, Transport and the Regions (DETR) is committed to working closely with people with learning disabilities and the transport industries to identify and meet the transport needs of people with disabilities. Government measures to improve access to transport for disabled people already taken or under way include:

- Implementation of the transport provisions in the Disability Discrimination Act;

- Development of disability training packages by the transport industry (supported by DETR);

- Greater emphasis on meeting the transport needs of disabled people, including those with learning disabilities, through Local Transport Plans;

- Increased focus on learning disability in the membership and agenda of DETR's Disabled Persons Transport Advisory Committee.

7.36 DETR will consult on proposals for legislation to outlaw discrimination against disabled people, including those with learning disabilities, on public transport and will monitor the effectiveness of local authority responses to meeting the needs of disabled people in the Local Transport Plans.

Leisure and Relationships

7.37 People with learning disabilities often do not take part in ordinary leisure activities. Leisure is rarely built into individual or community care plans. It tends to be seen as an optional extra, generally coming well down the list of agencies' priorities when decisions are being made about resources. Enabling people to use a wider range of leisure opportunities can make a significant contribution to improving quality of life, can help to tackle social exclusion, and encourage healthy lifestyles.

7.38 The Government expects local councils to ensure that their local cultural strategies and service plans encompass the needs of people with learning disabilities. This will include a review of physical

Heart'n'Soul – a national touring company of 10 people with learning disabilities and 4 professional musicians- was founded in 1986. It is based in the Albany Theatre London. The company has forged a name for itself on the international stage with performances. They run the Beautiful Octopus Club – a night club run and organised by people with learning disabilities. It has toured with 10 full scale musical productions and produced *Breaking the Rules*, its own half-hour television programme for BBC2.

access to leisure resources and ways to find out about them. Leisure will be an integral part of person-centred planning.

7.39 People with learning disabilities are often socially isolated. Helping people sustain friendships is consistently shown as being one of the greatest challenges faced by learning disability services. Good services will help people with learning disabilities develop opportunities to form relationships, including ones of a physical and sexual nature. It is important that people can receive accessible sex education and information about relationships and contraception.

Parents with a Learning Disability

7.40 The number of people with learning disabilities who are forming relationships and having children has steadily increased over the last 20 years. Parents with learning disabilities are amongst the most socially and economically disadvantaged groups. They are more likely than other parents to make heavy demands on child welfare services and have their children looked after by the local authority. People with learning disabilities can be good parents and provide their children with a good start in life, but may require considerable help to do so. This requires children and adult social services teams to work closely together to develop a common approach. Social services departments have a duty to safeguard the welfare of children, and in some circumstances a parent with learning disabilities will not be able to meet their child's needs. However, we believe this should not be the result of agencies not arranging for appropriate and timely support.

7.41 Support for disabled parents, including those with learning disabilities, is patchy and underdeveloped, as confirmed in the Social Services Inspectorate inspection *A Jigsaw of Services*[12]. There are tensions and even conflicts within social services departments between those whose focus is the welfare of the child and those concerned with the parent.

7.42 The Government's Framework for the Assessment of Children In Need and their Families is intended for use with all children in need and their families. Further work is needed to help staff use the Assessment Framework when working with parents with learning disabilities and ensure that assessments result in appropriate services being provided to the child and their family. The Department of Health will commission the development of training materials to

12 Department of Health, (2000) (CI (2000) 6) Social Services Inspectorate Inspection:
A Jigsaw of Services: Inspection of services to support disabled adults in their parenting role

assist in this process. Parents with learning disabilities will be a priority for follow-up work on the Assessment Framework. We shall also ensure that their needs and those of their children are addressed in future Quality Protects initiatives. The Department of Health will work with Sure Start and the National Parenting Institute to ensure that the needs of parents with learning disabilities are recognised within the Government's wider initiatives to improve parenting and family support.

7.43 At local level, it will be the responsibility of the Director of Social Services, as part of his/her responsibilities for ensuring quality under the social care Quality Framework to ensure effective partnership working for parents with learning disabilities between children's and adult's teams. Partnership Boards should ensure that services are available to support parents with a learning disability.

Social Security Benefits

7.44 For many learning disabled people, the social security system represents their main source of income. Only a small proportion are in paid employment and they are likely to be receiving benefits as well. The main benefits that learning disabled people receive are Income Support, Severe Disablement Allowance (SDA) and the Disability Living Allowance (DLA). They make up a significant proportion of the caseload for SDA (nearly a fifth) and DLA (10%).

7.45 A high proportion of decisions on DLA (Disability Living Allowance) are currently subject to successful challenge on appeal – around 46% for all cases and higher for cases involving some learning disabilities. The Government recognises the importance of ensuring consistency in decisions on entitlement. The Department of Social Security is developing a training programme for delivery to all staff, designed to lead to improvements in the quality of service provided to disabled people and their carers.

7.46 The Government is aware of concerns that attempting work or training will affect entitlement to DLA. Entitlement is assessed on a person's need for help with personal care and/or difficulty in getting round. People in work (see also paragraph 7.64) can receive DLA and evidence suggests that for many disabled people who work, this benefit provides important support. Indeed, some disabled people would not be able to work without the additional help and support provided by DLA.

7.47 Benefit decision makers are encouraged not to assume that starting work inevitably means that the severity of disabilities has reduced. Hard and fast rules are inappropriate, since some disabled people may require more support after starting work. The Department of Social Security has issued new guidance on this matter to benefit decision makers and is committed to keeping it under review. This should ensure that disabled people starting work do not lose their DLA without strong and sufficient reason. Complaints have reduced significantly since the guidance was improved.

7.48 The benefits system needs to keep pace with changes in society and the economy generally. The Government will shortly be introducing some changes to improve support for people with long-term sickness or disabilities, who rely on social security benefits:

- From April 2001, young people disabled before the age of 20, many of whom will have learning disabilities, will be able to qualify for Incapacity Benefit, without having to satisfy the normal contribution conditions. This age limit is extended to 25 for young people in education or work-based training immediately before the age of 20. From April 2002, these young people will get up to £27.60 a week extra from Incapacity Benefit (2001 benefit rates).

- A new premium in the income-related benefits will deliver, from April 2001, increased incomes for adults under 60 with severe disabilities and the greatest care needs who are on the lowest incomes. The Disability Income Guarantee will ensure an income of at least £142.00 a week for a single person and £186.60 for a couple. A new enhanced disability tax credit will be introduced to deliver equivalent increases within Working Families Tax Credit and Disabled Persons Tax Credit.

7.49 The Department of Social Security has a programme of work to help disabled people access benefits, including material for people who have difficulty using standard products. These are mainly targeted on clients who are visually impaired. It has also concluded that the best way to provide benefit information to people with learning disabilities and their carers is on a one-to-one basis. However the Department of Social Security plans to consult further about the most effective ways of communicating with people with learning disabilities and their carers to identify whether specially designed material would be effective.

MOVING INTO EMPLOYMENT

Government Objective: To enable more people with learning disabilities to participate in all forms of employment, wherever possible in paid work, and to make a valued contribution to the world of work.

7.50 The Government believes that employment is an important route to social inclusion and that all those who wish to work should have the opportunities and support to do so. Our Welfare to Work agenda is designed to increase employment opportunities for those who can work while retaining support for those who are unable to work. We will ensure that people with learning disabilities benefit from this major programme of reform.

Problems and Challenges

7.51 Disabled people are amongst those in our society with the lowest employment rates. It is likely that less than 10% of people with learning disabilities are in employment. Paid employment will not be a realistic option for all those with learning disabilities, but real jobs with real wages are a major aspiration for many people.

7.52 The reasons for this exclusion from the labour market are complex, but they include:

- Low expectations on the part of many agencies and professionals of what people with learning disabilities can achieve. This has meant that many learning disabled young people have not received training and preparation for employment. Services working with adults with learning disabilities have not seen helping them find work as a priority;

- The interaction between social security benefit rules and employment can result in disincentives to work for some learning disabled people;

- Difficulties in progressing from supported employment schemes (where these exist) into mainstream employment.

7.53 The Government is committed to helping more people with learning disabilities develop the skills they need to move into the labour market. Employment has the potential to improve people's financial situation, open up another source of friends and social contact and increase people's self-esteem.

What More Needs To Be Done

KEY ACTIONS – MOVING INTO EMPLOYMENT

- New Government target for increasing numbers of people with learning disabilities in work.

- New Workstep Programme will benefit people with learning disabilities.

- Joint Department of Health/Department for Education and Employment scoping study into links between supported employment and day services.

- Job Brokers under the New Deal for Disabled People will have skills in working with people with learning disabilities.

- Disabled people starting work will not lose Disability Living Allowance unfairly.

- Learning Disability Partnership Boards to develop local employment strategies.

- Better employment opportunities in public services for people with learning disabilities.

New Targets and Incentives

7.54 The Government's overall aim is to increase the number of people with learning disabilities in employment and to work towards their achieving parity with other disabled people in the workforce. Our target for this group is to increase the employment rate of people with learning disabilities and reduce the difference between their employment rates and the overall employment rate of disabled people. The challenge now is to ensure that our programmes and policies reach as many people with learning disabilities as possible and are delivered in ways which are responsive to their needs. The Government will work with the Employers Forum on Disability and the local Employer Networks to ensure that employers are engaged in this process.

7.55 The Government has taken a number of important steps to improve the incentives for moving into employment, including introduction of the minimum wage and the Disabled Person's Tax Credit which will help to achieve our target. We recognise that the interaction between benefit rules and income from employment can result in

Steven's Story

After Steven left school he went to an Adult Training Centre every day. By the age of 26 he felt ready to look for work. A trial work placement in a local garage was arranged. The owner realised Steven could locate and assemble parts into organised pre-assembly kits efficiently and accurately. Steven has now developed into a skilled and valued member of staff. 10 years later he is still working there on the assembly line with complex parts and production techniques.

disincentives for disabled people. Various measures have been introduced to address this, including:

- The improved Incapacity Benefit linking rule allows people to re-qualify for benefits if they move into work or employment training, but fall ill again and return to benefit within a year (two years if they move on to Disabled Persons Tax Credit);

- The higher earnings disregards in the Independent Living Fund for those of their clients who wish to work;

- From April 2001, the earnings disregard in income-related benefits will rise from £15 to £20 a week for disabled people and other special groups including carers.

Workstep: Reforming the Supported Employment Programme

7.56 Supported employment is provided by a variety of agencies including the voluntary sector, local authorities (usually via social services departments), and health authorities and through the Government's Supported Employment Programme. Many using supported employment are people with learning disabilities and in one form or another supported employment has traditionally been the main route to employment for people with learning disabilities.

7.57 A recent report by the Policy Consortium for Supported Employment takes stock of current provision and concludes that there is scope for considerable development in this sector. The report identifies barriers to the expansion of supported employment and proposes possible ways of tackling them.

7.58 The Government's Supported Employment Programme is operated by the Employment Service. Over 22,000 disabled people are employed at a cost of over £155 million including over 10,000 people employed by Remploy and over 12,000 people employed through Supported Employment Programmes (SEP) run by local authorities and voluntary bodies. Some 40% of those on SEP have learning disabilities – the highest single category of disability.

7.59 The Government is modernising the programme. From April 2001 it will be renamed Workstep and it will have greater focus on developing disabled people and helping them move into mainstream employment where they wish to do so and with longer term support available where needed. The aim for progression will be 10% a year for existing supported employees and 30% over two years for new supported employees. This figure may be adjusted once we have more information on which to base it. The evaluation of the programme will look at its impact on people with learning disabilities.

Links between Supported Employment and Day Services

7.60 The Government recognises that we need to look more closely at the interface between the full range of pre-vocational, employment and supported employment provision, including Department for Education and Employment's Workstep, and day services provided by local councils and the health service. The Department for Education and Employment and the Department of Health will establish a joint working group to explore this issue further, in partnership with local authorities and the voluntary sector. The two Departments will also jointly fund a scoping study to look at these issues in more depth. The outcome from this work will help the Learning Disability Partnership Boards in drawing up their plans to modernise day services.

The Working Age Agency

7.61 From summer 2001, the services currently delivered by the Employment Service and Benefits Agency will be brought together in the new Working Age Agency. This will allow for delivery of a more integrated and efficient service. It will be important that frontline staff in the new Agency have the right skills and training to work with people with learning disabilities. An appropriate training programme will be developed.

New Deal for Disabled People (NDDP)

7.62 The New Deal for Disabled People- the joint initiative between the Department of Social Security and the Department for Education and Employment – has been testing a range of approaches to find out how best to help disabled people who want to work. By the end of December 2000 the NDDP pilots had helped over 6,000 disabled people into work. NDDP will be extended nationally from July 2001, building on experience in the pilot phase. The development of a network of job brokers to offer work focused help to disabled people will be a central feature.

James's Story

James started working at Leeds United last season, a club for which he holds a season ticket. This is his first paid job, which means he can spend money on his other hobby- music. Before he had to save for weeks to buy CDs. When he started working, he received full training on which chemicals to use when cleaning and how to handle them. The training was tailor made so that he could recognise the different bottles easily. It was easiest for him to remember the pictures on the bottles and their colours. In the past people might say horrible things to James, which easily undermined his confidence. But he says that since he's been working it's really boosted his confidence. He's good at this job and so now has more responsibility overseeing different areas of work. He's made lots of friends since he started working, feels a sense of belonging and loves his job.

7.63 The Department for Education and Employment will ensure that the new job brokers have the skills needed to work with people with learning disabilities. Organisations bidding to be job brokers will need to have the right capacity and competences. Arrangements will be set up for sharing good practice and ensuring on-going strong performance by job brokers in this area. All organisations and individuals who work with disabled people must provide the support and advice they need to make appropriate decisions and be sensitive to the needs of people with learning disabilities. We will be looking to see what additional training and advice needs to be put in place.

The Disability Living Allowance (DLA)

7.64 As mentioned in paragraphs 7.46 and 7.47 this benefit provides important support for many disabled people who work. Disabled people in work can receive DLA and benefit decision makers are encouraged not to assume that starting work inevitably means that the severity of disabilities has reduced.

Local Employment Strategies

7.65 Local councils have been asked to have Joint Investment Plans for Welfare to Work for Disabled People in place by April 2001. This is an important tool for improving the range of local employment opportunities. In many areas, preparatory work for the Welfare to Work Joint Investment Plans has done a good deal to strengthen relationships between local councils and the Employment Service in order to increase employment opportunities for disabled people. The Government intends to build on these emerging links. Local Employment Services will be members of the Learning Disability Partnership Boards, and will play an active part in developing local employment strategies. These will include local targets for the employment of people with learning disabilities. Partnership Boards will also be expected to identify employment champions.

Better Employment Opportunities in the Public Sector

7.66 Central Government, local government and the NHS together form one of the largest employment groups in the world. A small minority within the public sector employ people with learning disabilities, but currently very few are employed in real jobs in either central or local government or the NHS.

7.67 The Government is committed to a dramatic improvement in diversity with the Civil Service, including the employment of disabled people. We will seek to improve our employment of people with learning disabilities as part of this process.

7.68 The Department of Health is committed to widening opportunities for employing disabled people, including those with learning disabilities, in the NHS. Local councils will be setting targets for the employment of socially excluded people, including people with learning disabilities, as part of Local Public Service Agreements.

CHAPTER 8

QUALITY SERVICES

8.1   The Government is committed to raising standards and improving quality in services for people with learning disabilities. Good quality services that promote independence, choice and inclusion will lead to good outcomes for people with learning disabilities. This chapter covers quality, workforce training and planning, resources and people with additional needs. The last topic covers services for people with profound and complex disabilities, people suffering from the autistic spectrum disorder; people with challenging behaviour, and people developing conditions associated with old age. These groups have additional and complex needs and achieving good quality services for them requires greater skill and effective co-ordination

QUALITY

Government Objective: To ensure that all agencies commission and provide high quality, evidence-based and continuously improving services which promote both good outcomes and best value.

Problems and Challenges

8.2   Quality assurance in learning disability services is currently underdeveloped. Few places have achieved a holistic approach that systematically draws on all sources of information and research, including feedback from users. Complaint procedures are often inaccessible. People from minority ethnic communities are too often at the margins of services and funding, and people with learning disabilities do not always receive adequate protection from abuse and exploitation. The challenge for agencies working in the learning disability field will be to:

- develop a better approach to measuring quality, which emphasises improved outcomes as informed by the best quality research;

- work in partnership with other agencies in developing benchmarks for measuring performance;

- enable people with learning disabilities to lead lives safe from harm and abuse;

- put the needs and wishes of the person using the service at the centre of their quality assurance systems.

What More Needs To Be Done

KEY ACTIONS – QUALITY

- National Minimum Standards for residential care for people with learning disabilities.

- Social Care Institute of Excellence to be leading source of expertise in learning disability informed by high quality research evidence base.

- Local quality assurance frameworks to be in place by April 2002.

- Department of Health guidance issued on user surveys in 2001.

- Local councils to collect information about incidents of abuse.

- DH guidance on physical interventions with people with learning disabilities in 2001.

- Measures to assist vulnerable or intimidated witnesses give evidence in court.

Care Standards Act 2000

8.3   The Care Standards Act 2000 introduces major changes to registration and inspection. It establishes a new regulatory framework for social care which will improve protection and raise standards for people with learning disabilities who use care services. The National Care Standards Commission (NCSC), which will come into operation from April 2002, will be responsible for ensuring that all regulated care services, including those managed by local councils, are provided to national minimum standards laid down by the Secretary of State. The Department of Health will be consulting on draft regulations and national minimum standards for care homes, adult placements and domiciliary services.

The Social Care Institute of Excellence (SCIE)

8.4 The Government is setting up the Social Care Institute of Excellence which will contribute to improvements in learning disability services by promoting evidence based practice to address the current variation in quality. The Department of Health will ensure that SCIE is properly equipped to become a leading voice in learning disability. SCIE will consult people with learning disabilities and their carers about guidelines on what works and produce their work in an accessible format.

Local Quality Frameworks

8.5 The new Quality Framework for Social Care – set out in *A Quality Strategy for Social Care* – and clinical governance in the NHS – set out in *A First Class Service* – together provide a means of promoting high quality services for people with learning disabilities. As part of their responsibilities under the Quality Framework, we expect Directors of Social Services to ensure that their local quality systems recognise and address the needs of people with learning disabilities. Given the importance of close integrated working for learning disability services, the Learning Disability Partnership Board will need to ensure the development of an integrated quality framework that applies across all agencies. This should make people with learning disabilities its central focus with their voices clearly heard and services clearly accountable to them.

8.6 An inter-agency quality assurance framework should be in place by April 2002.

User Surveys and Complaints Procedures

8.7 The Government expects people with learning disabilities and their carers to be fully involved in planning, monitoring and reviewing services; and also in evaluating the quality of the services they receive, as required under the new Quality Framework for Social Care. Local councils need to have a clearer picture of the experience of all users and carers who receive social care services, including hard to reach groups such as people with learning disabilities. The Department of Health will be issuing guidance in September 2001 to help local authorities improve the way they use and carry out surveys.

8.8 The Government believes that complaints procedures should be more accessible to service users and their carers. The Department of Health is currently considering ways of improving social services complaints procedures, including their accessibility. The NHS Plan commits the Government to reforming the NHS complaints procedures; the intention is to consult on proposals later this year.

Minority Ethnic Communities

8.9 The Government has identified many ways in which services and support to people with learning disabilities from minority ethnic communities are failing to meet the needs of individuals and their families. There are a small number of innovative initiatives across the country. These are not widespread and the Government expects all agencies to improve their practice to fulfil the objectives of the NHS Plan and legal obligations set out in the Race Relations (Amendment) Act 2000. Learning Disability Partnership Boards, which will largely be drawn from bodies which are subject to the new duty to promote race equality in the performance of their functions, should ensure that local services are culturally competent and can meet all the cultural needs of their communities.

Protecting Vulnerable Adults

8.10 People with learning disabilities are entitled to at least the same level of support and protection from abuse and harm as other citizens. This needs to be provided in a way which respects their own choices and decisions. Good quality services for people with learning disabilities must support them to lead lives safe from harm and abuse, whilst enabling them to lead fulfilling lives. The Department of Health's No Secrets guidance sets out a framework for the protection of all vulnerable adults that will provide important safeguards for people with learning disabilities. Local councils with social services responsibilities should take the lead in developing local policies and procedures for the protection of vulnerable adults within an inter-agency framework, which may be supported by the establishment of a multi-agency management committee.

8.11 Local councils will need to ensure that learning disability services are represented on local adult protection management committees, and that information about incidents of abuse of people with learning disabilities is gathered and recorded.

Imran's Story

Imran lives with his family, whose concerns for his welfare made them reluctant to introduce him to activities outside the home. Since becoming involved in a community-based group for Asian people with disabilities, he has grown in confidence and independent living skills. His family has developed more trust in what he can gain from an outside environment. Imran now has financial independence through his skills as an entertainer. He is often asked to perform at local and city-wide events and is a popular member of his community.

Vulnerable Witnesses

8.12 Although measures are in place to assist child witnesses, many adult victims and witnesses find the criminal justice process daunting and stressful. Some witnesses are not always regarded as capable of giving evidence and so can be denied access to justice. This can include people with learning disabilities.

8.13 In June 1998 the Government published the report *Speaking up for Justice*, which made 78 recommendations to assist vulnerable or intimidated witnesses, including children, give evidence in court and so improve their access to justice. Those recommendations requiring legislation were included in the Youth Justice and Criminal Evidence Act 1999 and will enable the court to order one or more of a range of measures to assist the witness in court. These include:

- screens round the witness box to prevent the witness viewing the defendant;

- giving evidence by live TV link;

- assistance with communication;

- video-recorded evidence in chief;

- use of an intermediary;

- video-recorded pre-trial cross-examination;

- clearing the public gallery in sex offence cases and cases involving witness intimidation.

8.14 The 1999 Act also amends the law on competency. This provides that as a general rule, all people, whatever their age, are competent to act as witnesses unless they cannot understand questions asked of them in court or cannot answer them in a way that can be understood, with, if necessary the assistance of any of the special measures above. The legislation also makes clear that those who are competent to give evidence but who are not allowed to give evidence on oath may give evidence unsworn. The Government is aiming to implement the majority of the special measures in the Crown Court by Spring 2002.

Physical Interventions

8.15 Many organisations and individuals are concerned about the inappropriate use of physical interventions with adults and children with learning disabilities. The Department of Health will be issuing guidance clarifying policy on the appropriate use of physical interventions later in 2001.

People with learning disabilities in prison

8.16 Prisoners with learning disabilities present a wide range of issues. The Prison Service seeks to identify their individual needs for education and health care within the framework of addressing their sentence requirements. Prison establishments have to balance the resources needed to deliver this level of care with the many other demands of prisoner management.

Resources and Best Value

8.17 The Government's aim is to ensure that people with learning disabilities gain fair access to, and maximum benefit from, all available resources, whether in mainstream services or specialist provision for people with learning disabilities. In order to achieve this, decisions about resource allocation need to be evidence-based and take account of the likely increase in demand for services from people with learning disabilities.

8.18 We know that expenditure on and costs of services for people with learning disabilities vary significantly from one authority to another. The scale of these variations is difficult to justify, and we believe that there is scope for the money currently devoted to learning disability services to be used more effectively. The application of Best Value principles will achieve better value for money. Many councils have chosen learning disability as an area for Best Value Reviews. To be most effective, such reviews will need to look at services from a whole systems perspective, rather than considering particular services, such as day services in isolation. They should be person-centred in their approach. Advice on designing such reviews will be available in 2001.

WORKFORCE TRAINING AND PLANNING

Government Objective: To ensure that social and health care staff working with people with learning disabilities are appropriately skilled, trained and qualified; and to promote a better understanding of the needs of people with learning disabilities amongst the wider workforce

Problems and Challenges

8.19 Implementing the Government's proposals will require a new focus on the skills and training of the social care and health workforce. While the data are not reliable, there may be as many as 83,000 people in the learning disability workforce (33,000 in local councils, 30,000 in the voluntary and independent sectors, 20,000 in the NHS). The problems for national Government, local agencies and individuals are:

- An estimated 75% of staff are unqualified;

- Difficulties in recruitment and retention of professional and care staff;

- Low status among the workforce;

- Few recognised accredited training qualifications;

- Little attention to workforce planning;

- Variable involvement of service users and carers in training or planning.

8.20 We need to be confident that people in this field are equipped to work in the new ways required by the new strategy. The challenge is to ensure that in future people working or dealing with people with learning disabilities are:

- Better trained and qualified with a commitment to lifelong learning;

- Skilled at working in partnership with users and carers;

- Confident in working in multi-professional teams, and across agency boundaries;

- Culturally competent;

- Part of a local workforce and services which represent their communities;

- Well led and managed.

8.21 People with learning disabilities come into contact with a wide range of other professionals in their daily lives: staff in social security offices, the Employment Service and housing agencies; teachers and lecturers; police; GPs and other staff in the NHS. All these groups would benefit from a wider understanding of the needs of people with learning disabilities so as to overcome any lingering prejudice and enable people to make use of services on an equal basis with other citizens. This is demanding but must be more than window dressing if the provisions of the Disability Discrimination Act are to be met.

What More Needs To Be Done

KEY ACTIONS – WORKFORCE

- Health and Social Care Workforce Strategies to provide new opportunities for learning disability staff.

- Learning Disability Awards Framework introduced in April 2001.

- Learning Disability Development Fund to support range of leadership initiatives.

- Local Workforce Planning and Training Plans.

Health and Social Care Workforce Strategies

8.22 The Government has set in train major changes to lifelong learning and training. The Learning and Skills Council with its Local Learning Partnerships are expected to promote opportunities for education and lifelong learning, which will help develop a knowledge based approach in the workforce. The Department for Education and Employment's scheme to establish Individual Learning Accounts (ILAs) will help individuals meet the costs of training. The Government has set out general workforce strategies for health and social care which offer new opportunities for the learning disability field. The new Quality Framework for Social Care recognised the need for a new focus on workforce training and development. The NHS Plan promises all staff receiving dedicated vocational training – including those working in the learning disability field – a £150 individual learning account to 'top up' the contribution from the Department for Education and Employment scheme.

8.23 The Training Organisation Personal Social Services (TOPSS) National Training Strategy (endorsed by Government) contains specific proposals about learning disability. In 2001/2002 £2 million is being provided for TOPSS to support implementation of the Training Strategy. TOPSS will use the funds to roll out training based on the new Induction Standards for social care staff. TOPSS Regional Forums will administer this funding.

8.24 In each area the new NHS Workforce Confederations will involve all service providers- health, social care, independent and voluntary. TOPSS Regional Training Forums should work together with the Confederations to maximise the impact of training for staff in all sectors. The Confederations will have increased capacity to consider local workforce demands in learning disability. The Government will ensure that the work of each Confederation takes full account of the proposals set out here.

Learning Disability Awards Framework (LDAF)

In Bristol Social Services and Health we already provide a structured programme of training on issues such as 'Protecting Vulnerable Adults' and 'Working with Challenging Behaviour'. LDAF is what we've been waiting for – a framework which will give staff a nationally recognised qualification for all the learning they have done. Because of the new Awards, staff will be motivated to think more about their own development, and there will be close links with the NVQ level 3, which will all help towards creating a better qualified workforce. This will benefit the people who use our services – which is really what the whole thing is about!

Bristol Social Services and Health

8.25 The Government recognises that the levels of skills, training and qualification in the learning disability workforce need to be raised. We are therefore introducing from April 2001 a new Learning Disability Awards Framework, within the existing qualifications structures, to provide a recognised route to qualification and career progression for care workers in learning disability services. By April 2002 all new entrants to learning disability services will be registered for the new awards. The Framework is based on two new vocational qualifications:

● A level 2 Certificate in working with people with learning disabilities;

● A level 3 Advanced Certificate in working with people with learning disabilities.

Government Targets

From April 2002 all new entrants to learning disability care services should be registered for qualification on LDAF.

By 2005 50% of front line staff should have achieved at least NVQ level 2.

8.26 The new qualifications provide a comprehensive summary of learning outcomes, mapped against occupational standards. The new Framework will enable staff and employers to plan career paths and provide a route for people to progress to higher education and professional qualifications.

8.27 In partnership with TOPSS we have set some ambitious targets for rollout of the Framework. These will be monitored through data collected from the awarding bodies, National Open College Network and City and Guilds Affinity.

8.28 The next phase of the work on LDAF is in hand to bring levels 4 and 5 into the Framework. The General Social Care Council comes into operation in October 2001. The Department will explore with the Council how the Learning Disability Awards Framework can be linked to registration requirements for the learning disability sector.

Involving Users and Carers

"I want staff who treat you well, who know how to treat you properly"

8.29 The best way to achieve this is to promote the involvement of people with learning disabilities and their family carers in training and development activities. Staff and managers at all levels in organisations need to have an opportunity to hear directly from people with learning disabilities about their expectations. Some authorities have already begun to enable service users to play an effective role in the design and delivery of training to both managers and front-line staff.

Leadership

8.30 Effective leadership is essential for achieving the changes required. The Government will use the Learning Disability Development Fund to support a range of initiatives aimed at enhancing professional and managerial leadership in learning disability services. As part of the programme of work to implement this White Paper, we will also:

- Further develop the leadership capacity of people with learning disabilities and carers;

- Work in partnership with elected local councillors who have an important role to play in promoting positive acceptance of people with learning disabilities by the wider community;

- Recognise the valuable role to be played by academic leadership in creating and developing appropriate learning systems, stimulating investment in applied research and teaching and encouraging a new generation of leaders.

Wendy's Job

Wendy has a job teaching health care staff. *'Teaching Doctors about Disability is very powerful and I enjoy it, but am exhausted afterwards. Getting the job in the first place was very difficult, I was lucky I had the right support, but it was really, really hard and I had to do a lot of preparation before I started!'*

Local Workforce Plans

8.31 Learning Disability Partnership Boards will be required to develop a workforce and training plan. These should cover how service users and carers are being involved in training and workforce matters, the content and quality of health professional training, resourcing training and development needs across all organisations in the field including the independent sector and proposals for dealing with any shortfall in staffing.

People with Additional and Complex Needs

8.32 Good quality services will ensure that people with additional and complex needs are appropriately cared for so that their needs are well managed and they lead fulfilling lives. This includes people who:

- have severe and profound disabilities (including those with sensory impairments);

- have epilepsy;

- have an autistic spectrum disorder and also a learning disability;

- present with behaviour that challenges their carers and service providers;

- develop conditions associated with old age.

People with severe and profound disabilities

8.33 People with severe and profound learning disabilities often have other associated health problems such as physical disabilities, sensory impairments and epilepsy. They will almost always require a greater level of health care support than is usually available from a primary health care team. Members of the specialist learning disability service should provide additional support to the primary health care team to help them manage the complex health needs of those with multiple disabilities. In addition they may need access to a range of medical, nursing and other health services including physiotherapy, occupational therapy, speech and language therapy and orthopaedic services. Those who are technology dependent will require substantial additional support. The numbers of children who are technology dependent are relatively small, but an increasing number are surviving into adulthood.

Margaret's Life

Margaret lived almost all her life in largish homes with people she didn't particularly enjoy being with. She acquired neither language nor formal signing, but was very well able to make her wishes known. She lost contact with her family once her mother died, but acquired a long-term personal advocate who gave her links with the outside world and helped her do some of the things she enjoyed: meals out, long walks, her own personal holiday. This was the one person who was "there for her", and the advocate was with her during her last days and when she died.

8.34 People with profound and complex disabilities may have difficulty communicating their needs and wishes. They may need the support of someone who knows them well such as a family member, an advocate or a supporter. Nevertheless, it is important to enable people with profound and complex needs to exercise as much control as possible over their own lives.

People with epilepsy

8.35 The rate of 'active' epilepsy for people with mild or moderate learning disabilities is 5% compared to a normal rate of 0.5% in the general population. We may expect to find 30% of people with severe learning disabilities at risk of developing epilepsy, rising to 50% among those with profound learning disabilities. The condition originates in childhood for the majority. For people with Down's syndrome the onset of seizures in middle age may be associated with the onset of dementia.

8.36 Modern diagnostic investigations include referral to a specialist with expertise in epilepsy for detailed examination. People with severe and profound disabilities may have difficulties in co-operating with the investigations and specialist neurological clinics may be reluctant to accept such referrals. All people with learning disabilities are entitled to have access to specialist clinics, including tertiary services. Adequate and appropriate facilitation must be available to enable this to happen. Good support of the person with epilepsy involves careful and sympathetic understanding, effective monitoring of medication and support of daily routines to minimise the impact of factors that may provoke seizures.

People with learning disabilities and autistic spectrum disorders

8.37 Many people with severe and profound learning disabilities have autistic behaviours, even if not formally recognised. It is important that all services for people with learning disabilities have the skills to recognise and make adequate provision locally for them although the majority will not need autism specific services. The presence of an autistic disorder is normally first recognised in early childhood. The diagnosis depends on a full and competent assessment from a child and adolescent psychiatric, paediatric or learning disability service that specialises in this area. A number of new diagnostic instruments have recently been introduced and are currently being evaluated.

8.38 Many parents face lengthy waiting times for early diagnosis of autistic spectrum disorders. This often reflects the high workload of child development centres and Child and Adolescent Mental Health services and a lack of skilled expertise in diagnosing autistic spectrum disorders. This is in part being addressed by a joint initiative by the Department of Health and Royal College of Psychiatrists to develop a training programme for paediatricians with special expertise in mental health disorders.

8.39 The Department of Health has asked the Medical Research Council to obtain a clear and comprehensive picture of current knowledge about the incidence, prevalence and causes of autism and the strength of the evidence which underpins that knowledge. The Medical Research Council will submit a report to the Department of Health in autumn 2001. This will be circulated more widely to a range of policy-makers, patients, interest groups, the research community and the public.

8.40 Recent research suggests that family based early intervention for children with autistic spectrum disorders may result in improvements in skill and behaviour. Early intervention helps a significant number to overcome their disability sufficiently to attend mainstream schools. However, throughout their lives the majority of people with autistic spectrum disorders require educational, social, psychological and therapeutic interventions. Real choice is often limited by what is available rather than what might best suit the individual, and referral to residential services far from home is not uncommon. The Government will continue to work with the relevant professional bodies and other experts on autism to consider how screening, diagnosis and early intervention can be improved.

8.41 Although we focus on the needs of those individuals with autism who have learning disabilities, some general principles apply. Children with autism are children first and their needs as children should be the main focus. Whether or not they have learning disabilities in addition to their autism, they should therefore benefit from our proposals for improving services for disabled children.

8.42 Adults with autism need a range of living and working environments. Those who require intensive treatment and support are often unable to access local services and are referred to residential services far from home. While this may suit some individuals, others may prefer to live in their local community, take part in a local day service, find a job or seek supported employment. Person-centred planning should make it possible for individuals to be able to exercise their choice in how their housing and support is provided.

People with learning disabilities who have challenging behaviour

8.43 Commissioning and providing services for people who present significant challenges is one of the major issues facing learning disability services. The presence of challenging behaviour does not make an individual the responsibility of the NHS, although the NHS is responsible for commissioning and providing appropriate health input including intensive support from health professionals. The report of the Mansell Committee (Department of Health 1993) provided guidance on this and stressed that services should be commissioned on an individualised basis and should seek to promote inclusive lifestyles.

8.44 Challenging behaviours are best thought of as being a way in which people respond and try to gain control over difficult situations. Sometimes the challenging behaviour may be triggered by pain and a full medical assessment should always be undertaken. Psychotropic medication may be very effective when there is an underlying psychiatric disorder but there is concern that too often this medication is used as an alternative to adequate staffing. Modern behavioural approaches can result in significant short and medium term reductions in the severity of the behaviour. Learning Disability Partnership Boards should ensure that local services develop the competencies needed to provide treatment and support within the local area. To facilitate this, we have made developing specialist services for people with severe challenging behaviour and/or autism one of the priorities for the capital element of the Learning Disability Development Fund.

Older people with learning disabilities

8.45 Many people with learning disabilities now in their 50s and 60s were not expected to outlive their parents. Improved medical and social care now means they are living longer. Life expectancy is influenced by the severity of the learning disability. Those with severe and profound disabilities tend to die younger. As with the rest of the population women survive longer than men. Many of those now entering old age have spent most of their lives in long-stay hospitals and are likely to be adjusting to a new life in a home of their own, in supported living or in a small group home. A small number have continued to be in the care of the NHS in continuing care provision.

8.45 There are some people with learning disabilities over the age of 75, who have shown significant physical and mental deterioration with age, who have high dependency needs and who make considerable demands on health and social services. Their difficulties as older people overshadow any problems associated with their learning disability and their needs are practically identical to those of the elderly population as a whole. Person-centred plans for these individuals should be developed in the context of services for elderly people.

8.46 There are other older people with learning disabilities who are more mentally alert and have aspirations more typical of younger people. They may be misplaced in older peoples' homes living alongside much older and more incapacitated people. Plans for these individuals should be developed around packages of occupational and recreational activities and residential support which takes account both of their learning disabilities and the ageing process. They should be enabled to be as actively engaged as possible.

8.47 Those who develop Alzheimer's disease have very special needs. About a third of those with Down's syndrome may be expected to show clinical evidence of dementia, but others without Down's syndrome may also develop dementia. In Down's syndrome the onset of dementia may be from 35 years of age or earlier and their health often deteriorates quite rapidly. Providing good quality support for these individuals is a major challenge. The Government will expect learning disability services to work with the specialist mental health services to ensure that, between them, appropriate supports are provided for younger people with learning disabilities suffering from dementia.

8.48 The NSF for Older People will set out a framework that applies to services for all people over 65 years of age. But for people with learning disabilities the ageing process may begin much earlier. This means that planning for the needs of "older people" with learning disabilities may need to include a more extended population, perhaps taking account of those aged from 50 years upwards. Developing the person-centred approach to planning services described in Chapter 4 will enable local agencies to address the needs of older people with learning disabilities. Local Partnership Boards will ensure that there is co-ordination between learning disability services and older people's services so that people can access the services which are most appropriate to their needs.

PART THREE:

DELIVERING CHANGE

CHAPTER 9

PARTNERSHIP WORKING

Government Objective: To promote holistic services for people with learning disabilities through effective partnership working between all relevant local agencies in the commissioning and delivery of services.

9.1 This objective aims to promote:

- **Rights:** local Partnership Boards will need to ensure the availability of service options to meet people's assessed needs and wishes;

- **Independence:** agencies responsible for mainstream housing, education, employment and leisure will be fully included in local planning and commissioning;

- **Choice:** greater integration between agencies will open up wider service options for all people;

- **Inclusion:** people with learning disabilities and their families will be given the opportunity to be involved in local partnerships.

This objective is concerned with services for adults, with partnership for children services continuing to be addressed through Children Services Plans.

Problems and Challenges

9.2 Effective partnerships are key to achieving social inclusion for people with learning disabilities. Learning disability services have traditionally shown innovative approaches to partnership working. However, these are not widespread for reasons including:

- A lack of agreement about values and service objectives;

- An inability or unwillingness to agree on financial arrangements;

- Low priority being given to joint working within organisations.

9.3 In many places, people with learning disabilities and their families continue to be passed between organisations and professionals with insufficient clarity about where responsibility rests for ensuring effective service provision. Community learning disability teams were forerunners in partnership working, but they have not consolidated their position.

9.4 People with learning disabilities and their families need to have confidence that all organisations are working together to achieve integrated service planning and commissioning, and that they can gain access to their choice of services through one clear access route.

What More Needs To Be Done

KEY ACTIONS: PARTNERSHIP WORKING

- Learning Disability Partnership Boards to be established by October 2001.

- National support to partnership working to be provided through the Learning Disability Development Fund, Implementation Support Team and the production of good practice advice.

- Partnership Boards to agree plans for the use of Health Act flexibilities in the updated Joint Investment Plan (JIP).

- Further Department of Health guidance on partnership working and future role of community learning disability teams.

Partnership Boards

9.5 The Government intends to build on existing inter-agency planning structures to establish Learning Disability Partnership Boards in all local authority areas by October 2001. Partnership Boards will be responsible for those elements of the Government's proposals which relate to services for adults with learning disabilities. Services for disabled children will continue to be addressed through children services planning structures. The Partnership Board will operate within the overall framework provided by Local Strategic Partnerships (LSPs).

9.6 The development of Local Strategic Partnerships (LSPs) offers a framework for local partnership working, bringing together public, private, community and voluntary sectors in order to provide effective co-ordination. These arrangements aim to simplify and expand the scope of partnerships concerned with community well-being. Many areas already have a strategic partnership on which an LSP can build. Our proposals for partnership working in learning disability will fit within the overall umbrella offered by LSPs. Close links between Learning Disability Partnership Boards and LSPs will ensure a common direction and help to address wider issues, such as access to other local services, including transport.

9.7   Learning Disability Partnership Boards will not be statutory bodies. They will be responsible for:

- Developing and implementing the Joint Investment Plan for delivering the Government's objectives;

- Overseeing the inter-agency planning and commissioning of comprehensive, integrated and inclusive services that provide a genuine choice of service options to people in their local community;

- Ensuring that people are not denied their right to a local service because of a lack of competence or capacity amongst service providers;

- The use of Health Act flexibilities;

- Ensuring arrangements are in place to achieve a smooth transition to adult life for learning disabled young people.

9.8   Learning Disability Partnership Boards should particularly ensure that:

- people with learning disabilities and carers are able to make a real contribution to the Board's work;

- the cultural diversity of the local community is reflected in its membership;

- local independent providers and the voluntary sector are fully engaged.

9.9   It will be the responsibility of the chief executive of the local council to ensure that the Partnership Board is in place. Membership should include senior representatives from social services, health bodies (health authorities, Primary Care Trusts (PCTs)), education, housing, community development, leisure, independent providers, and the employment service. Representatives of people with learning disabilities and carers must be enabled to take part as full members. Minority ethnic representation will be important in view of the Government's commitment that their needs should not be overlooked.

9.10 The Learning Disability Development Fund and Implementation Support Team will make partnership development an early priority. The Department of Health will issue further guidance on partnership working in 2001.

Health Act Flexibilities

9.11 The new flexibilities introduced by the Health Act 1999 (see glossary) already provide opportunities to improve partnership working. They also provide the framework within which Learning Disability Partnership Boards will be required to operate. The NHS Plan makes clear that the Government expects the partnership flexibilities to be used in all parts of the country. Some localities are making early use of these flexibilities in the learning disability field, and we believe that wider use of these flexibilities will benefit people with learning disabilities and their families.

9.12 The Government expects all agencies involved in the Partnership Boards to show in their updated JIPs that they have fully considered how to use the Health Act flexibilities to underpin effective partnership working.

9.13 Joint Investment Plans will be evaluated and monitored to ensure effective partnership working. Evidence of failings in partnership arrangements will be taken into account in determining the allocation of the new Learning Disability Development Fund. Where there is evidence that services for people with learning disabilities are failing, partnership working is unsatisfactory and the Health Act flexibilities not being properly used, the Government will consider use of the new powers of intervention contained in the Health and Social Care Bill, which will enable the Department to direct the use of the partnership arrangements.

9.14 The Government places emphasis on the importance of promoting choice and achieving inclusion for people with learning disabilities through close partnership between health and social services and a wide range of other agencies including employment, education, housing and the and voluntary and independent sectors. In this context, it is likely that the leadership of the local partnership will rest with the local council, making use of one or more of lead commissioning, joint commissioning and pooled budgets.

Cumbria County Council, Morecambe Bay Health Authority, and North Cumbria Health Authority have agreed to commit £20 million to a pooled fund for learning disabilities. The intention is to enable an integrated strategy to be delivered, providing a consistent and high quality service, which can respond to the needs of individuals. The Partnership Arrangement has been established on the basis of broad participation from users, carers, providers – statutory and independent. It has clear performance measures based on priorities identified through the consultation process – including improving respite care, day care and activities, and reducing the size of accommodation units. Lack of co-terminosity has not been a barrier to development. A project manager has been appointed who is focusing on where integrated provision would enable the strategy to be fulfilled.

9.15 However, where effective partnerships are not established with local council leadership, the Government will consider using its intervention powers to require the development of a Care Trust. There may also be particular local circumstances which make the creation of a Care Trust an appropriate way to achieve local integration of services.

The Role of Primary Care Trusts (PCTs)

9.16 Primary Care Trusts (PCTs) will be key players in the Learning Disability Partnership Boards. As PCTs become more firmly established and develop their commissioning responsibilities, they will be the lead health body for learning disability services. They will need to develop skills and knowledge in commissioning learning disability health services. Partnership Boards will not constrain the freedom of emerging PCTs, but will enable them to enhance the effectiveness of their overall contribution to improving health outcomes for people with learning disabilities.

Integrated Professional Working

9.17 Professional structures need to ensure that people with learning disabilities and their families have easy access to services from all agencies. To achieve this, Partnership Boards should review the role and function of community learning disability teams in order to ensure that:

- All professional staff become accountable for the outcome of their work to the local partnership arrangements – whilst ensuring the retention of appropriate professional accountabilities and support;

- All professional staff become a resource for the local implementation of the White Paper and to help achieve social inclusion for people with learning disabilities;

- Organisational structures encourage and promote inclusive working with staff from the fields of housing, education, primary care, employment and leisure.

9.18 The Department of Health guidance on partnership working will provide further advice on the future role of community teams.

CHAPTER 10

MAKING CHANGE HAPPEN

10.1 Delivering the Government's ambitious plans for people with learning disabilities will take time, as real change always does. Improving the lives of people with learning disabilities is a complex process which requires a fundamental shift in attitude on the part of a range of public services and the wider local community. This will not be easy. It needs real leadership at both national and local levels, supported by a long-term implementation programme with dedicated resources and on-going action to monitor delivery. This chapter sets out how the Government intends to approach this challenging task.

10.2 The Department of Health in partnership with the Department for Education and Employment, the Department of the Environment, Transport and the Regions and the Department of Social Security will issue further guidance on what is expected of local agencies in order to implement the new strategy.

National Action

Learning Disability Task Force

10.3 The Government will set up a national Learning Disability Task Force to take forward the implementation. The role of the Task Force will be to monitor and support implementation by acting as a champion for change and improvement at local level. Drawing on the knowledge and experience of members, the Task Force will also offer advice to Government on the continuing development of learning disability policy. It will focus on the adult elements of the Government's proposals, and its membership will be drawn from a wide range of interests, including minority ethnic communities. The Children's Task Force will continue to have the lead on disabled children's issues and we will ensure that effective links are in place between the two.

10.4 People with learning disabilities and carers will be full members of the Task Force. We will ensure that effective links are in place between the Task Force and the National Forum for People with Learning Disabilities.

Learning Disability Development Fund

10.5 To support implementation of the new proposals for adults, the Government will create a new Learning Disability Development Fund of up to £50 million per annum, of which up to £30 million will be revenue funding and £20 million capital. This will be introduced in April 2002 and will be targeted on the Government's priorities.

10.6 The revenue element of the Development Fund will be created from that element of the current old long-stay adjustment within general health allocations which is released as former long-stay patients die. We will conduct a census of old long-stay patients through the NHS regional offices later in 2001 in order to determine the final size of the Development Fund. We will announce this in good time before April 2002.

10.7 The Development Fund will be used to support our priorities for service change. Priorities for the use of revenue funding will be:

- Modernising day centres;

- Completing the reprovision of the remaining long-stay hospitals to enable people to move to more appropriate accommodation by April 2004;

- Developing supported living approaches for people with learning disabilities living with older carers;

- Promoting the further development of advocacy;

- Supporting the wider introduction of person-centred planning;

- Enhancing leadership in learning disability services.

10.8 Priorities for the use of the capital will be:

- enabling local providers to develop specialist services for people with severe challenging behaviour;

- developing integrated health and social services facilities for children and young people with severe disabilities and complex needs;

- developing supported living approaches for people with learning disabilities living with older carers.

10.9 Learning Disability Partnership Boards will be required to submit updated Joint Investment Plans (JIPs) to the Department of Health by January 2002, setting out their plans for implementing the White Paper. Updated JIPs should include bids against the capital element of the Learning Disability Development Fund. Decisions about the allocation of the Learning Disability Development Fund will require the social care and health regions of the Department of Health to be satisfied that the JIPs are acceptable and that in particular they provide evidence of satisfactory partnership arrangements.

10.10 The Learning Disability Development Fund will be made available subject to the condition that the resources may only be used where they are deployed as part of pooled funds under the Health Act flexibilities. This will enable the Learning Disability Development Fund to support the implementation of all aspects of *Valuing People*. Learning Disability Partnership Boards will be required to show how they will make use of the Health Act flexibilities to enhance partnership working and this will be taken into account in decisions about the allocation of the Development Fund.

Implementation Support Team

10.11 We believe that a strong national lead which provides effective support to local action will be vital in delivering the vision set out in *Valuing People*. The Government will therefore set up a national Implementation Support Team during 2001. The team will be led by a Director with a Development Worker based in each of the eight Department of Health regions and will be charged with promoting good practice and sharing practical experience across the country.

Implementation Support Fund

10.12 The Government will set up an Implementation Support Fund of £2.3 million a year for 3 years from April 2001 to provide central support for key aspects of the new strategy. (This includes £300,000 for increasing volunteering opportunities for citizen advocates.) Priorities for the Fund include:

● Development and expansion of advocacy services;

● Establishment of a National Learning Disability Information Centre and Helpline in partnership with Mencap;

- Funding a number of development projects on key priorities, including person-centred planning, partnership working and a scoping study of the interface between employment and day services;

- Extension of the Learning Disability Awards Framework.

Improving the Information Base

10.13 National data on learning disability issues are currently underdeveloped. The Government intends to take steps to improve the situation. During 2001/02, the Department of Health will commission a national survey of people with learning disabilities in contact with social services in order to improve our knowledge and provide a stronger baseline against which to evaluate the impact of *Valuing People*.

10.14 The Department of Health will also be undertaking a project to improve its own data collection in the learning disability field by establishing which activities and services should be the subject of regular statistical returns. For disabled children, the children in need census is already improving the knowledge base, and the forthcoming Integrated Children's System will set out the minimum data requirements for collecting information about individual children and families, including disabled children.

Research

10.15 Research has an important role to play. Findings from research contribute towards fostering an evidence based approach to service delivery. The Department of Health will be funding a £2 million research initiative *People with Learning Disabilities: Services, Inclusion and Partnerships* starting in 2001/02 and lasting for four years. The areas we wish to study are:

- Service delivery in health and social care and its effectiveness to identify elements of good practice, implementation and sustainability;

- Social inclusion, including access to good health care, and the factors which create disability barriers in people's lives;

- Organisation development to show how staff performance in learning disability services can be supported to achieve better services.

10.16 The aim of this initiative is to generate a knowledge base to inform the implementation of our proposals. We expect to fund 6–10 studies. The initiative will be overseen by a reference group and its findings disseminated to complement the *Valuing People* implementation programme.

10.17 There is already a considerable amount of research activity on learning disability in the NHS. Over 130 separate research projects, as listed on the National Research Register (NRR), have recently been completed. About £3 million is being spent on 50 current studies. Topics being researched include the health needs of people with learning disabilities in the community. Among those recently completed were a study of women with learning difficulties and their experiences of cervical smear tests and research on the impact of training for carers, on the mental health of people with learning disabilities.

10.18 The NHS Information Authority will develop a National Electronic Library for Learning Disability. In 2001/2002 the Authority will be putting more resources into the pilot project.

Inspection

10.19 We shall ensure that the Social Services Inspectorate (SSI) and the Commission for Health Improvement (CHI) give attention to learning disability services within their national work programmes. During 2001/02, there will be a national inspection by SSI of learning disability services in order to assess how well placed local councils will be to implement the new strategy. Findings from the inspection will be used to inform the work and priorities of the Implementation Support Team.

Local Action

10.20 Learning Disability Partnership Boards will be accountable for implementing the proposals in *Valuing People* at local level. Boards will be expected to appoint a senior officer who will have lead responsibility for taking this forward.

10.21 Health and local authorities have already been asked to have learning disability Joint Investment Plans (JIPs) in place by April 2001. Guidance on the development of the learning disability JIP foreshadowed some of the key themes in the new strategy. The Government has therefore decided to build on the JIPs as the basis for local implementation of its proposals. Learning Disability

Partnership Boards will be required to develop local action plans as supplements to the JIP and to submit the updated JIP to the regional offices of the Department of Health by 31 January 2002. The JIPs will then be jointly evaluated by Department of Health social care and NHS regional offices.

10.22 As part of overall guidance on implementation, the Department of Health will issue guidance on the contents of the updated Joint Investment Plan (JIP). It will be essential that the JIP is agreed by all agencies represented on the Learning Disability Partnership Board. The Government will expect people with learning disabilities, carers and the local voluntary and independent sectors to be fully involved in this process.

Delivery Plan

10.23 Set out below are the key actions which will be taken by the Government and by local agencies to implement the new strategy. This needs to be at least a five year implementation programme. Although we are clearer now about the early milestones, the Learning Disability Task Force will revisit this plan on a regular basis to roll it forward for future years.

Spring 2001

- Recruitment of Implementation Support Team begins
- Funding for Citizen Advocacy Network and Self-Advocacy work comes on stream
- Work begins in partnership with Mencap to develop National Information Centre
- Regional office census of former old long-stay patients carried out
- Guidance on person-centred planning commissioned
- Guidance on Physical Interventions issued
- All new entrants to learning disability care services should be registered on LDAF

Summer 2001

- Learning Disability Task Force established

- Issue guidance on implementation

- Issue joint DH/DETR guidance on housing for people with learning disabilities

- DH/DfEE study into interface between day services and supported employment commissioned and DH/DfEE joint working group set up

- Work under way to establish National Learning Disability Users Forum

Autumn 2001

- Implementation Support Team up and running

- Guidance on direct payments issued

- Good practice materials on learning disabled people and decision making issued

- Good practice materials on partnership issued

- Learning Disability Partnership Boards in place

- Issue guidance on person-centred planning

Winter 2001/02

- Learning Disability Partnership Boards submit updated JIP to the Department of Health which is to act as local action plan

- Complete analysis of JIPs and notify decisions about Learning Disability Development Fund

Spring 2002

- Introduction of new Learning Disability Development Fund

- Agree local framework for person-centred planning and begin implementation

- Inter-agency framework for quality assurance to be agreed

- Plans for closing remaining long-stay hospital units agreed

Winter 2002/03

- Day service modernisation programme agreed
- JIP updated
- Agree Housing Strategy
- Agree Employment Strategy

Summer 2003

- All Learning Disability Partnership Boards to have agreed framework for Health Action Plans
- Health facilitators identified.

Winter 2003

- Person-centred planning for people in long-stay hospitals completed.
- Full range of employment and support service options in place

Targets post March 2004

- Programme to enable people still living in long-stay hospitals to move into more appropriate accommodation by April 2004
- 50% of front line staff to have achieved at least NVQ level 2 – 2005
- All people with a learning disability to be in receipt of a HAP by June 2005
- Modernisation of day centres completed by 2006

Monitoring Delivery

10.24 Delivering the changes set out in *Valuing People* involves a complex range of agencies, including at least four Government departments and a wide range of local agencies. The large number of stakeholders involved makes it particularly important that the Government takes a comprehensive approach to monitoring implementation. We will ensure that existing performance assessment mechanisms across health, social services, education, employment and housing enable us to monitor implementation of the key initiatives. Best Value and the performance assessment arrangements for social services are likely to make a particularly important contribution, given the lead role that local councils have in taking forward our proposals.

10.25 We have reviewed the existing data and performance indicators which are already in place on learning disability services, and are proposing new performance indicators for use as part of the further development of JIPs. These are set out at Annex A in support of the Government's objectives for learning disability services. We intend to replace the existing national performance indicators within the social services Performance Assessment Framework with new outcome-focused indicators. We shall consult Local Government Association, Association of Directors of Social Services and the NHS Confederation on more detailed proposals.

Conclusion

10.26 We do not underestimate the difficulties involved in delivering our ambitious new vision for people with learning disabilities. The principles of rights, independence, choice and inclusion we put forward are challenging and have far reaching implications for all those agencies – public, independent and voluntary – who work with people with learning disabilities. Enabling people with learning disabilities to have their voices heard and have wider opportunities for a fulfilling life as part of the local community is central to our message. Delivering this involves new ways of working in more effective partnerships. But getting it right for people with learning disabilities will show what can be achieved with and for one of the most vulnerable and socially excluded groups in our society.

ANNEXES

OBJECTIVES AND SUB-OBJECTIVES, TARGETS AND PERFORMANCE INDICATORS

Objective 1: Disabled children and young people

To ensure that disabled children gain maximum life chance benefits from educational opportunities, health care and social care, while living with their families or other appropriate settings in the community where their assessed needs are adequately met and reviewed.

BY:

Sub-objective 1.1
Ensuring early identification of disabled children to enable them to access appropriate and timely intervention and support

Sub-objective 1.2
Ensuring that parents and disabled children receive reliable, comprehensive and culturally appropriate information about services on a multi-agency basis from the statutory and voluntary sectors.

Sub-objective 1.3
Increasing the number of disabled children in receipt of a range of family support services and the number of hours provided.

Sub-objective 1.4
Maximising the number of children with disabilities/special educational needs who receive good quality co-ordinated care and education in inclusive settings in their own communities.

Sub-objective 1.5

Ensuring that disabled children receive appropriate health care throughout childhood so as to enable them to participate fully in education, family and community life.

Sub-objective 1.6

Increasing the number of disabled children who use inclusive play, leisure and cultural services including holiday play schemes, after schools clubs and pre-school provision with appropriate support if necessary.

Performance against this objective and associated sub-objectives will be measured through the Quality Protects programme

The above sub-objectives build on existing Government Objectives for Children's Social Services and will be finalised in the autumn Quality Protects circular

Objective 2: Transition into adult life

As young people with learning disabilities move into adulthood, to ensure continuity of care and support for the young person and their family, and to provide equality of opportunity in order to enable as many disabled young people as possible to participate in education, training or employment.

BY:

Sub-objective 2.1

Ensuring that each Connexions partnership provides a full service to learning disabled young people by identifying them, deploying sufficient staff with the right competencies and co-ordinating the delivery of appropriate supports and opportunities.

The Connexions Unit headline target for young people at risk (including people with learning disabilities) is: participation and achievement over time to converge with those in the population in the same age group

Sub-objective 2.2

Ensuring effective links are in place within and between children's and adult's services in both health and social services.

Objective 3: More choice and control

To enable people with learning disabilities to have as much choice and control as possible over their lives through advocacy and a person-centred approach to planning the services they need.

BY:

Sub-objective 3.1

Promoting the rights of people with learning disabilities

Sub-objective 3.2

Enabling advocacy to be available for people with learning disabilities who want or need it.

Proposed Performance Indicator and PAF Indicator: The amount spent by each council on advocacy expressed as the amount per head of people with learning disabilities known to the council

Sub-objective 3.3

Making direct payments available to all those people with learning disabilities who request them and who meet the requirements of the scheme.

Proposed Performance Indicator: % of people with learning disabilities receiving community based services who are receiving direct payments

Sub-objective 3.4

Developing locally agreed protocols and procedures to ensure services are based upon a person-centred approach.

Sub-objective 3.5

Ensuring that people with learning disabilities are fully and actively involved in all decisions affecting their lives.

Objective 4: Supporting carers

To increase the help and support carers receive from all local agencies in order to fulfil their family and caring roles effectively.

BY:

Sub-objective 4.1
Assessing the needs of carers and putting in place the services required.

Proposed Performance Indicator: % of adults with learning disabilities receiving community based services who are receiving short term breaks

Sub-objective 4.2
Establishing a complete picture of the number of older carers (ie those aged 70 and over) in the local area in order to plan services in partnership with them.

Proposed Performance Indicator: % of carers aged 70 or over for whom a plan has been agreed

Sub-objective 4.3
Providing services and support that meet the needs of carers from minority ethnic communities.

Sub-objective 4.4
Making sure that all agencies work in partnership with carers, recognising that carers themselves have needs which must be considered.

Objective 5: Good health

To enable people with learning disabilities to access a health service designed around their individual needs, with fast and convenient care delivered to a consistently high standard, and with additional support where necessary.

BY:

Sub-objective 5.1
Reducing the health inequalities experienced by people with learning disabilities.

Sub-objective 5.2

Enabling mainstream NHS services, with support from specialist learning disability staff, to meet the general and specialist health needs of people with learning disabilities.

Sub-objective 5.3

Promoting the development of NHS specialised learning disability services which are evidence based and delivered with a focus on the whole person.

The Department of Health will develop performance indicators to compare the health status of people with learning disabilities with that of the general population and will consult on these.

Objective 6: Housing

To enable people with learning disabilities and their families to have greater choice and control over where, and how, they live.

BY:

Sub-objective 6.1

Increasing the range and choice of housing open to people with learning disabilities in order to enable them to live as independently as possible.

PAF PERFORMANCE INDICATOR: B14 Unit Cost of residential and nursing care for adults with learning disabilities

Sub-objective 6.2

Ensuring people with learning disabilities and their families obtain advice and information about housing from the appropriate authorities.

Sub-objective 6.3

Enabling all people currently in NHS long-stay hospitals to move into more appropriate accommodation and reviewing the quality of outcomes for people living in NHS residential campuses.

Target: Enabling the people currently living in NHS long-stay hospitals to move to more appropriate accommodation by April 2004

Objective 7: Fulfilling lives

To enable people with learning disabilities to lead full and purposeful lives within their community and to develop a range of friendships, activities and relationships.

BY:

Sub-objective 7.1

Modernising day services to enable people to exercise real choice over how they spend their days

Proposed Performance Indicators:

- **Gross expenditure on day care as a percentage of expenditure on all non-residential services**

- **Ratio of expenditure on day and domiciliary services for people with learning disabilities to expenditure on residential provision for people with learning disabilities**

Sub-objective 7.2

Enabling people with learning disabilities to have access to a wide range of opportunities for education and lifelong learning in order to promote greater independence and maximise employment opportunities.

The Learning Skills Council (LSC) will set targets as part of its equal opportunities strategy

Sub-objective 7.3

Enabling people with learning disabilities to make full use of transport and access mainstream community and leisure services.

Sub-objective 7.4

Supporting parents with learning disabilities in order to help them, wherever possible, ensure their children gain maximum life chance benefits.

Sub-Objective 7.5

Making sure that people with learning disabilities receive the social security benefits to which they are entitled.

Objective 8: Moving into employment

To enable more people with learning disabilities to participate in all forms of employment, wherever possible in paid work and to make a valued contribution to the world of work.

BY:

Sub-objective 8.1
Ensuring that more people with learning disabilities find appropriate employment, including supported employment, which makes the most of their talents and potential.

Proposed National Target: Increase the employment rate of people with learning disabilities and reduce the difference between their employment rates and the overall employment rate of disabled people

Proposed Performance Indicator: number of people with learning disabilities in work as a proportion of those with learning disabilities known to the council

Sub-objective 8.2
Making sure that people with learning disabilities are actively helped to access employment related advice and guidance through mainstream and specialist advisory services.

Sub-objective 8.3
Ensuring that public services provide a lead in the employment of people with learning disabilities.

Objective 9: Quality

To ensure that all agencies commission and provide high quality, evidence based, and continuously improving services which promote both good outcomes and best value.

BY:

Sub-objective 9.1
Demonstrating that people with learning disabilities and their families are increasingly satisfied with services provided.

Sub-objective 9.2
Ensuring that the needs of people with learning disabilities from minority ethnic communities are recognised and addressed through the provision of appropriate services.

Proposed Performance Indicator: the proportion of people with learning disabilities from minority ethnic communities who are receiving services divided by the proportion of all people in the local population from minority ethnic communities

Sub-objective 9.3
Ensuring that local quality assurance frameworks for social care and health meet the needs of people with learning disabilities.

Sub-objective 9.4
Ensuring people with learning disabilities receive best value from publicly funded services.

Proposed Performance Indicator: Number of people with learning disabilities known to the local council per head of general population

Sub-objective 9.5
Ensuring that local adult protection policies and procedures (including those for protecting vulnerable victims and witnesses of crime) are in place and fully complied with.

Objective 10: Workforce and planning

To ensure that social and health care staff working with people with learning disabilities are appropriately skilled, trained and qualified; and to promote a better understanding of the needs of people with learning disabilities amongst the wider workforce.

BY:

Sub-objective 10.1
Introducing the new national framework for training, competencies, qualifications and skill levels in the learning disability workforce.

Targets

- **From 2002 all new entrants to learning disability care services to be registered with Learning Disability Awards Framework**

- **By 2005 50% of front line staff to have achieved at least NVQ Level 2**

– **Proposed Performance Indicator: Percentage of staff working in learning disability services achieving at least NVQ Level 2**

Sub-objective 10.2
Promoting awareness among the wider workforce (in areas such as housing, the wider NHS, transport and the Department of Social Security) of the skills, attitudes and knowledge needed to work with people with learning disabilities in a positive and respectful manner.

Sub-objective 10.3
Ensuring that local workforce plans are developed.

Objective 11: Partnership working

To promote holistic services for people with learning disabilities through effective partnership working between all relevant local agencies in the commissioning and delivery of services.

BY:

Sub-objective 11.1
Establishing local Learning Disability Partnership Boards to take responsibility for local delivery of the White Paper, led by the local council and with the active participation of all key stakeholders.

Target Date: October 2001

Sub-Objective 11.2
Making effective use of the Health Act flexibilities.

Sub-objective 11.3
Promoting effective partnership working by staff from all relevant disciplines and agencies.

The Department of Health will be consulting further with the Local Government Association, the Association of Directors of Social Services and the NHS Confederation on the proposed indicators and consequential changes to the PAF Indicators. The agreed set of indicators will then be used to assess performance in the supplements to JIPs required by January 2002.

The Department of Health will be commissioning a national survey of people with learning disabilities in order to improve knowledge about the lives of people with learning disabilities and their families. It is anticipated that fieldwork would begin towards the end of 2001/2002.

GLOSSARY

Childcare Development Partnerships – *aim is to establish good quality affordable childcare in all communities. From 2001 all will be required to identify and train a special educational needs (SEN) co-ordinator.*

Children's Fund – *£450 million Government programme targeted at preventive work with vulnerable children (primarily in the 6 to 13 age group). Strong emphasis on voluntary sector delivery.*

Connexions Service – *brings together into a single strategy across Government policies for young people aged between 13 and 19. Provides advice and support, gives particular attention to those at greatest risk of not making a successful transition to further leering and adulthood.*

Direct payments – *cash payments service users can receive from social services departments to purchase for themselves services to meet their assessed needs. The only service they cannot be used for is permanent residential care.*

Disability Rights Commission – *set up following recommendations from the Disability Rights Task Force and the Disability Rights Commission Act 1999 to work towards the elimination of discrimination against disabled people. Came into operation April 2000.*

Health Act flexibilities – *provisions in the Health Act 1999 enabling local authorities to work more closely with health authorities to provide improved services.*

Intentional community – *services operated by independent sector organisation comprising houses and some shared facilities on one or more sites and based on philosophical or religious belief.*

Joint Investment Plans (JIPs) – *plans produced jointly by local authorities, health authorities, and other local stakeholders for the integrated provision of services for a range of client groups.*

Learning and Skills Council – *set up under the Learning and Skill Act 2000. Has overall responsibility for post-16 education below higher education.*

Learning Disability Advisory Group – *set up in 1998 to advise Ministers on issues affecting people with a learning disability. Members include professionals, NHS and LA representatives, voluntary organisations, researchers, service users, and parents.*

NHS residential campus – *service operated by an NHS Trust comprising housing, some of which will be clustered on one site, together with some shared central facilities and developed as a direct result of the closure of NHS hospitals.*

NHS Plan – *contains proposals for ensuring that health services more fully meet the needs of patients.*

Old long-stay patients – *patients with a learning disability who were admitted to hospital prior to 1 January 1970 and who were still receiving care on 1 April 1996.*

Quality Protects – *Government programme designed to improve children's social services.*

Reprovisioning – *developing alternative settings for services currently or formerly provided in long-stay hospitals, large hostels, day centres etc.*

Sure Start – *Government programme aimed at promoting the physical, intellectual, and social well-being of pre-school children.*

Village communities – *service operated by independent sector organisation comprising houses clustered on one site together with some shared central facilities.*

ANNEX C

BIBLIOGRAPHY

This lists some of the main publications which informed the development of *Valuing People*.

Abott, David: Morris Jenny, and Ward, Linda, (2000) *Disabled Children and Residential Schools; a Study of Local Authority Policy and Practice* Norah Fry Centre

Ahmad, Waqar, (2001) Centre for Research in Primary Care, University of Leeds, *Learning Difficulties and Ethnicity*

Association for Residential Care (1999–2000) *Training Networks Research*

Brown, Hilary, (2000) *Abuse and protection issues*, Centre for Applied Social and Psychological Development, Canterbury Christ Church University College

Chamba, Rampaul, et al, (1999) *On the Edge: Minority Ethnic Families Caring for a Severely Disabled Child*, Policy Press

Department for Education and Employment (1998), *Meeting Special Educational Needs: A Programme for Action*

Department for Education and Employment (2000), *Connexions: the Best Start in Life for Every Young Person*

Department of Health (1992) (Chairman: Prof. J L Mansell) *Services for People with Learning Disabilities and Challenging Behaviour or Mental Health Needs.*

Department of Health (Circular HSG (92) 42) Health Services for People with Learning Disabilities (Mental Handicap)

Department of Heath (Circular LAC (92) 15) *Social Care for Adults with Learning Disabilities* (Mental Handicap)

Department of Health, (1997) *People Like Us: The Report of the Review of the Safeguards for Children Living Away from Home*

Department of Health (1998) *Moving into the Mainstream: The Report of a National Inspection of Services for Adults with Learning Disabilities*

Department of Health (1998), *Signposts for Success in Commissioning and Providing Health Services for People with Learning Disabilities*

Department of Health (1998) *Disabled Children; Directions for their Future Care*

Department of Health (1999) *Once a Day*

Department of Health (1999) *Facing the Facts: Services for People with Learning Disabilities: Policy Impact Study of Social Care and Health Services*

Department of Health, (2000) *A Jigsaw of Services: Inspection of services to support disabled adults in their parenting role*

Department of Health, Department for Education and Employment, Home Office (2000) *Framework for the Assessment of Children in Need and their Families*

Department for Education and Employment, National Training Organisation (1997) *Learning and Working Together*

Emerson, Eric, (2000) *Challenging Behaviour: Analysis and Intervention in Intellectual Disabilities*, Cambridge University Press

Glendinning, Caroline, and Kirk, Sue,(1999) *The Community-Based Care of Technology Dependent Children in the UK: Definitions, numbers and costs*, National Primary Care research and Development Centre, University of Manchester

Gordon, David, Parker, Roy, Loughran, Frank, (2000) *Disabled Children in Britain, a re-analysis of the OPCS Disability Surveys*, the Stationery Office

Hester Adrian Research Centre, University of Manchester (1999), *Quality and Costs of Residential Supports for People with Learning Disabilities – Summary and Implications*

Local Government Management Board: (1999) *Recruitment Trends* (1999) *Recruitment & Qualifying WF* (1998) *SSD Qualifying WF/WF* (1997) *Human Resources for Personal Social Services*

Mencap (2000) *Learning Disability Strategy Initial Submission*

Mencap, (2000) *New targets for a new century: learning disability strategy*

Morris, Jenny, (1999) *Hurtling into the Void*, Pavilion Publishing,

Morris, Jenny, (1998) *Still Missing? The experiences of disabled young people living away from their families*, The Who Cares? Trust

NHS Cancer Screening Programmes (2000) *Good Practice in Breast and Cervical Screening for Women with Learning Disabilities*

NHS Executive (2001), *From Words Into Action: The London Strategic Framework for Learning Disability Services*

O'Bryan, Anne, Simons, Ken, Beyer, Steve, Grove, Bob, (2000) *A Framework for Supported Employment*, Joseph Rowntree Foundation

Russell, Philippa, (1998) Council for Disabled Children *Having a Say! Disabled Children and Effective Partnership in Decision Making*

Saving Lives: Our Healthier Nation. The Stationery Office (ISBN 0-10-143862-1)

Ward, Cally, *(2001) Family Matters, Counting Families In:* The report from the Family Carers working group

The six working groups listed in Annex D considered papers prepared by their members on a range of subjects.

ADVISORY GROUPS AND WORKING GROUPS

Learning Disability Advisory Group

Ann Gross, Disability Branch, Department of Health (Chair)

Colin Beacock – Royal College of Nursing
Norma Brier – Norwood Ravenswood
Maurice Brook – Rescare
James Churchill – Association for Residential Care
Jean Collins – Values into Action
Yvonne Cox – NHS Confederation
Ian Davey – Association of Directors of Social Services
Eric Emerson – Institute for Health Research (Lancaster University)
Rob Greig – Community Care Development Centre
John Harris – British Institute of Learning Disabilities
Fred Heddell – Mencap
Sheila Hollins – St George's Hospital Medical School
Mary Lindsey – Royal College of Psychiatrists
Joan Maughan* – National Development Team
Bill Robbins – Association of Directors of Social Services
Noel Towe – Local Government Association
Jan Webb – Success in Shared Care
Chris Wells – Department for Education and Employment

* replaced Simon Whitehead

Department of Health officials:
  Catherine Baines – Disability Branch
  Alistair Brechin – Disability Branch
  Sue Carmichael – Nursing Division
  Elaine Cooper – Disability Branch
  David Ellis – Inspector, Disability Branch
  Patricia Parris – Disability Branch
  Oliver Russell – Senior Policy Adviser (Medical), Disability Branch

Services Users Advisory Group*

Change:
Paul Adeline
Mary Byrne
Andrew Gayle
Justine March
Jean Sapsford

Mencap:
John Atkinson (died February 2001)
James Calvert
Mabel Cooper
Jenny Green
Margaret Perks

People First:
Michael Brookstein
Michelle Chinnery
Andrew Lee
Carol Lee
Raymond Johnston
Eve Rank-Petruziello
John Watson

Supporters
Tim Gunning
John Herzov
Andrew Holman
Penny Mendonca

* Representatives from the Service Users Advisory Group are also full
members of the Learning Disability Advisory Group

Working Groups

Children

Catherine Baines – Department of Health (Joint Chair)
Peter Smith – Department of Health (Joint Chair)
Shobha Asar-Paul – Birmingham Social Services Department
Gillian Batt – Department of Health
Jayne Boyfield – Department of Health
Norma Brier – Norwood Ravenswood
Richard Carter – Department of Health
Susan Clarke* – Department for Education and Employment
Eric Emerson – Institute for Health Research (Lancaster University)
Ruth Fasht – Norwood Ravenswood
Ann Gross – Department of Health
Philippa Russell – Council for Disabled Children
Kim Sibley – Department for Education and Employment
Linda Ward – Rowntree Foundation

*replaced Kim Sibley

Carers

Cally Ward – Independent Consultant (Chair)
Tim Anfilogoff – Department of Health
Cathy Baines – Department of Health
Joan Barnard – Success in Shared Care
Ruth Bayard – Norwood Ravenswood
Peter Scott Blackman – The Afiya Trust
Maurice Brook – Rescare
Sue Carmichael – Department of Health
Richard Kramer – Mencap
Robina Mallet – Home Farm Trust
Joan Maughan – National Development Team
Philippa Russell – Council for Disabled Children
David Thompson – Mental Health Foundation
Carol Walker – Sheffield Hallam University

Health

Oliver Russell – Department of Health (Joint Chair)
Sue Carmichael – Department of Health (Joint Chair)
Ann Barwood – Department of Health
Jean Collins – Values into Action
Yvonne Cox – NHS Confederation
Ronnie Croft – Department of Health
Mark Davies – Department of Health
Roger Deacon – Social Services Department, Surrey County Council
Margaret Flynn – National Development Team
Pauline Fox – Department of Health
Ann Gross – Department of Health
Jacqui Howard – Department of Health
Nick Harris* – Department of Health
Sheila Hollins – St George's Hospital Medical School
David Ockelford – Department of Health
David Towell – Community Care Development Centre

*replaced Jacqui Howard

Supporting Independence

Ann Gross – Department of Health (Chair)
Jane Ashworth – Department for Education and Employment
Catherine Baines – Department of Health
Michael Brookstein – People First
Michelle Chinnery – People First
David Ellis – Department of Health
Gwylfa Evans – Association of Directors of Social Services
Jacqui Howard-Department of Health
Carol Lee – People First
Michael Lloyd – Department of Social Security
Brian McGinnis – Mencap
Barbara McIntosh – Community Care Development Centre
Hester Ormiston – Department of Health
Martin Routledge* – Department of Health
Jim Sherwin – Department for Education and Employment
Ken Simons – Norah Fry Research Centre
David Towell – Community Care Development Centre
Frances Walker – Department of the Environment Transport
    and the Regions
Zoe Wentworth – Department of Health
Simon Whitehead – National Development Team

*replaced Jacqui Howard and Hester Ormiston

Workforce Planning and Training

Sue Carmichael – Department of Health (Joint Chair)
David Ellis – Department of Health (Joint Chair)
Richard Banks – TOPSS England
Colin Beacock – Royal College of Nursing
Colin Bott – Department of Health
Sally Burton – Department of Health
James Churchill- Association for Residential Care
Jennifer Lyon – Department of Health
Joan Maughan – National Development Team
Debbie Mellor – Department of Health
Anne Mercer – Department of Health
David Mellor – Improvement and Development Agency
Francis Ward – TOPSS England

Building Partnerships

Rob Greig – Social Care Group, Department of Health (Chair)
Carole Bell – Department of Health
Colin Bott – Department of Health
James Churchill – Association for Residential Care
Elaine Cooper – Department of Health
Michael Lloyd – Department of Social Security
Janice Miles – NHS Confederation
Bill Robbins – Association of Directors of Social Services
Wendy Wallace – Department of Health
Jan Webb – Success in Shared Care

Printed in the UK for The Stationery Office Limited
on behalf of the Controller of Her Majesty's Stationery Office
05/03   65536   ID 142855
Reprinted 2003